conception
& pregnancy
over 35

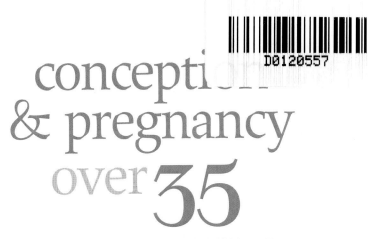

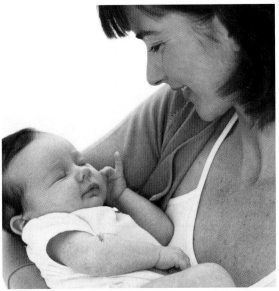

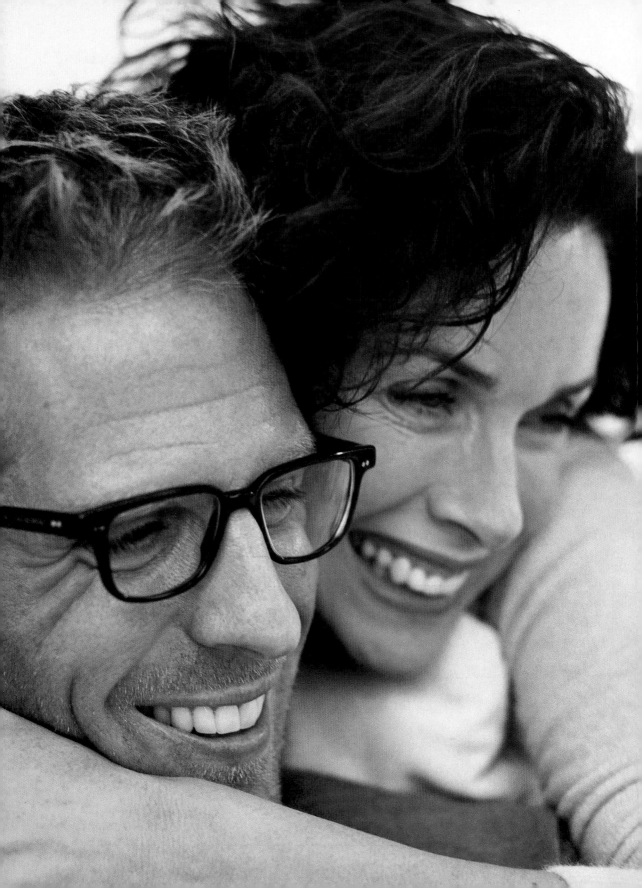

conception
& pregnancy
over 35

Dr Laura Goetzl

and Regine Harford

LONDON, NEW YORK, MUNICH,
MELBOURNE, DELHI

Senior editor Janet Mohun
Art editor Sara Kimmins
Designer Alison Turner
DTP designer Julian Dams
Picture research Samantha Nunn
DK picture librarian Romaine Werblow
Illustrator Debbie Maizels
Production controller Luca Frassinetti
Managing art editor Emma Forge
Art director Carole Ash
Publishing manager Anna Davidson
Publishing director Corinne Roberts

First published in Great Britain in 2005 by
Dorling Kindersley Limited,
80 Strand, London WC2R 0RL
A Penguin Company

A CIP catalogue record for this book is available
from the British Library

ISBN 1 4053 0639 4

Reproduced by Colourscan, Singapore
Printed and bound in Singapore by Star Standard

see our complete catalogue at
www.dk.com

contents

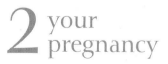

3 adjusting to motherhood

foreword

It is always a pleasure to read a new book about pregnancy that offers something different and successfully addresses a previously unmet need. Dr Goetzl has produced a book that specifically addresses the concerns and needs of women over 35 who want to become pregnant, stay pregnant and go on to have a healthy baby. It is a timely addition to the bookshelves as the number of babies born in the UK to women over the age of 35 has more than doubled during the last decade and now represents around 1 in 6 of all births. Similar maternity statistics can be found for women in the US and Europe.

As a fertility doctor, I am impressed by the sensible but sensitive advice offered in the first section of the book, which deals with preconception planning, problems conceiving, assisted conception, and miscarriage. Importantly, we are reminded that conceiving in the late 30s will probably, but not necessarily, take a bit longer and that most couples are successful eventually. This is a refreshingly upbeat approach – given that the media tend to focus on women with reproductive difficulties.

As a practising obstetrician caring for women who have had problems in previous pregnancies (who tend to be older), I am pleased to see comprehensive information on antenatal screening and tests. The explanations offered on fetal monitoring in pregnancy and the practicalities of labour and delivery will also be warmly received. Finally as an older mother myself, it is refreshing to see that issues such as increased fatigue during pregnancy and the possibility of a longer time being needed to recover postnatally have not been glossed over. All in all, this is a timely and useful book that will provide the growing number of women over the age of 35 with the additional reassurance and confidence that they need to enjoy a successful pregnancy.

Professor Lesley Regan MD, FRCOG
Head of Department of Obstetrics and Gyneacology
St Mary's Hospital, Imperial College, London

introduction

When I started to think about writing this book, I soon realized there was a real need for information specifically geared for women considering pregnancy somewhat later in life, especially for first-time mums. Women often feel there is pressure to have children early, yet more and more are waiting to conceive, delaying motherhood to establish their career, meet their ideal partner, or start a second family.

As women mature, their circumstances change, as does the way they approach motherhood. You are more likely to be college-educated, in a stable relationship, and more proactive about gathering information on your pregnancy. At the same time, somewhat arbitrarily, as a woman over 35 you are placed in a "high risk" category by the health professionals looking after you and possibly even by your friends and family. Medically, this high-risk status means you will be offered more tests and more information to decipher than younger women. Emotionally, you may find you have more decisions to make and more unsolicited advice to field.

With all of this in mind, Regine Harford and I have sought to write a book that addresses your concerns and seeks to reaffirm and reassure. We aim to empower you with information

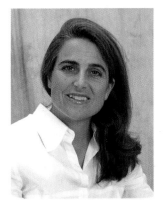

that will allow you to step into one of the most important roles of your life with self-assurance. I want this book to give you the confidence to face the normal difficulties of pregnancy and early motherhood believing that you know what is best for yourself as an individual, and what is best for your baby. I hope you find this this book is helpful to you and provides you with the support you need. Enjoy!

Dr. Laura Goetzl

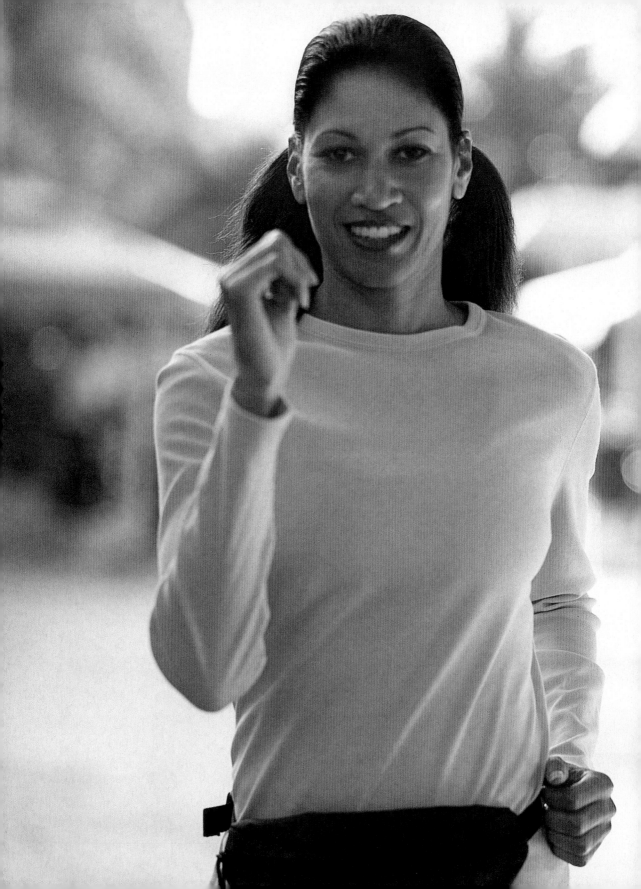

PLANNING FOR CONCEPTION

MANY WOMEN FIND **CONCEIVING** AFTER AGE 35 IS NOT AS EASY AS THEY THOUGHT IT WOULD BE. LOOKING AFTER YOURSELF, BY **EATING WELL** AND KEEPING FIT, CAN HELP **BOOST FERTILITY**. SOME PROBLEMS WITH FERTILITY ARE A DIRECT RESULT OF **MEDICAL CONDITIONS** THAT ARE MORE LIKELY AS YOU GET OLDER. SPENDING TIME **GETTING INFORMED** BEFORE YOU CONCEIVE IS REALLY WORTHWHILE. IF YOU DO HAVE PROBLEMS **BECOMING PREGNANT**, THERE ARE MANY THINGS **YOU CAN DO** TO HELP AND IF ALL ELSE FAILS **ASSISTED CONCEPTION** MAY BE THE ANSWER.

making the decision

Pregnancy is the first step in a life-changing and life-long relationship with your child. Becoming a parent can be one of the most gratifying and joyful aspects of your life, but it requires you to invest much of your time, money, and emotional resources. Therefore, the decision to become pregnant should come only after thoughtful consideration of some important facts.

WHEN IS THE RIGHT TIME?

Many couples want to wait for the perfect time to have a baby – a time when material, professional, and relationship conditions are flawless. But career, financial, and health challenges can arise at any time. Thankfully, babies thrive in imperfect conditions, so neither you nor your circumstances need to be perfect.

Some women have always wanted to be mothers, while others look at babies with ambiguity. If your interest in motherhood is recent, you may wonder whether life with a baby is for you. For many women in their 30s and 40s who have built rich, fulfilling lives, some uncertainty about becoming a mum is natural.

You may have a lot invested in your career, partnership, and friendships, and have hobbies and activities that are close to your heart. Pregnancy will require major changes in your lifestyle, as will motherhood. You will have to care for your child at all times of the day, resulting in a significant loss of freedom and spontaneity in your life that can be very difficult to accept, especially if you have enjoyed a great degree of independence up to now.

Spending time with friends who are parents is good preparation for parenthood as it gives you a realistic view of the challenges involved.

HAVING A REALISTIC OUTLOOK

Smiling mums caring confidently for their cute babies are the staple of advertisements aimed at parents-to-be. The reality of uncountable sleepless nights, crying infants, and the frustration of not knowing what's wrong with your baby are rarely mentioned. Babies are demanding and unpredictable. They can't tell you

ARE YOU READY FOR PARENTHOOD?

■ How is your emotional and physical health?

A cranky or sick baby and sleepless nights can drain your energy, especially if you have health problems. But making sure that you get enough rest and some regular time away from your baby can help to preserve your strength.

■ Do you have experience with children?

Babies can go from a big smile to a heart-wrenching scream in a split second and without an obvious reason. If you have never cared for a young child, you may often feel out of control when you become a mum. Spending some time with mums and their babies can help you develop confidence in your child-caring abilities.

■ Is parenting a priority for you and your partner?

Your pregnancy and the arrival of your baby will disrupt the time you and your partner have together. If one of you is significantly less committed to becoming a parent, ongoing baby needs can become a point of contention. Having a reliable, flexible childcare arrangement and good support from family and friends can keep your relationship on track.

■ How much of your energy goes into your career?

Having a baby can feel like taking on a second job. If you have a stressful career that requires long hours, you may find there is not enough time and energy to do both jobs well. Consider how you might be able to adjust your working life to allow for baby care.

■ Can your recreational activities include a child?

Babies require regular meals, nappy changes, and safe places to sleep. If ski slopes, kayaks, art museums, or lecture halls are among your favourite recreational places, adjusting your hobby and finding a fun babysitter for your child may help create an acceptable balance between your social life and time spent with your child.

■ Are you financially prepared for parenthood?

You and your partner should consider all the financial aspects of bringing up children, such as the costs of childcare, clothes, toys, and practical equipment such as pushchairs and car seats, then plan your post-baby finances accordingly. Ask friends who are parents for information.

what they need, which can make you feel lost and out of control, a feeling you might not enjoy, particularly if you take pride in being organized and efficient. Babies are also time-consuming and command attention on their terms rather than yours. If they are hungry or uncomfortable, or if they just want to be cuddled, they will let you know and stop crying only after you have guessed their needs. Your baby will become your first priority for a while and this can put a serious strain on your relationships, impact upon your career, and shake up your self-image as a capable, independent person.

However, often the aspects of our lives that demand the most attention are also the ones we come to cherish as the most worthwhile and enriching. Your baby will not only turn your world upside down, he or she will also teach you about your immense capacity to nurture life. Your baby will return your

love, making you feel like the most special person in the world. That aspect of motherhood can make it feel like the best job on earth. Even in the most frustrating moments as a parent, a smile or big, bright grin from your baby can make you forget your exhaustion and the missed opportunities to be with your friends.

PRECONCEPTION CARE

Emotional and physical readiness for pregnancy is especially important for mature mums-to-be, because they significantly affect your fertility, your wellbeing during pregnancy, and your baby's health. During pregnancy your body will meet your baby's needs before your own, so stacking your physical and emotional resources to optimal levels now will prevent depletion of your strength during pregnancy and speed up your recovery after birth.

your relationships

Fertility is reduced with age, and conception times for mature couples are longer (see pp24–25). Don't let a few months of waiting make you and your partner feel inadequate, which can lead to discord in your relationship. One important aspect of preconception care therefore is making sure that you feel hopeful and remain emotionally balanced.

LOOKING AFTER YOURSELF

The monthly ritual of counting down to your optimal conception days and then waiting for the time of your next period can deplete your emotional energy. There are various strategies you can use to help you and your partner maintain an equilibrium.

Devising a monthly routine Because the waiting phase may last many months, you may want to devise the least elaborate monthly routine acceptable to you and your partner. It is best to decide on just one method to assess your fertile days and make sure that it feels natural and simple to you. For some women the temperature/mucus method works, others use an ovulation calculator on their computers and mark

reassure your partner of his **essential role** in your life

their calendars accordingly (see pp24–25). Stick to just one method. Using several at once may lead to an obsessive preoccupation with conception.

Finding compassionate support After repeated unsuccessful attempts to become pregnant, feelings of disappointment and inadequacy can dominate your thoughts. You may wonder whether you will be able to conceive at all. Sharing these emotions with

women who have gone through the preconception phase or are currently doing so can be reassuring and the advice and support you receive can bring back your positive outlook. Relevant support groups for women over 35 can be found on the internet and in your local community. Alternatively, you might consider seeing a professional counsellor.

BECOMING A PARENTING TEAM

Your partner will bring his hopes and fears to the process of becoming a parent. Traditionally, mothers have been the primary caretakers of children, especially during infancy, and many men fear that their wife's love will be diverted completely to the baby. It's always good for both of you to discuss your feelings and remember that your relationship as a couple is really important and that you don't lose sight of this in your attempts to start a family.

Commitment to parenthood In an ideal world, both partners in a relationship are equally committed to the process of a planned conception and pregnancy. However, it may sometimes be necessary for the more committed partner to make concessions to reward the reluctant partner's investment of time and effort. A partner may feel happier if, for example, you could move closer to extended family for practical help or if he could have a regular night out with friends.

Coping with planned sex If you are having any problems or delays in conceiving, you might get to the point where you really need to plan when you have sex to optimize the chances of conceiving. Try not to let the idea of scheduling sex put a strain on your relationship. Instead, make the idea of a "sex date" exciting rather than boring. Leave a suggestive note in his pocket or diary. Use these times to put aside your everyday concerns and focus on your partner. Also, remember you don't have to restrict lovemaking to these times of the month. Take care to focus on the pleasure of being with your partner while having sex rather than on becoming pregnant.

Your monthly waiting cycles The monthly wait to see whether you menstruate, and sharing another "failure to conceive", can leave you and your partner feeling emotionally drained. Plan for a fertility holiday when you are not "trying" to get pregnant. Agree on a number of monthly cycles (perhaps once every 4–6 months) where your mind will not be occupied with conceiving. You may plan special times away from home during these weeks and allow yourselves an emotional respite.

On Your Own

Single parenting may raise some eyebrows – being a trail blazer is never easy. You may have chosen IVF or perhaps decided not to marry the man who will father your baby. You are not alone. More and more women choose not to settle for unsatisfying partnerships in order to have a baby. But they still build especially close relationships with their children. A good support network is vital. This network should include a compassionate and capable medical team who treat your body gently, and respond to your questions thoughtfully and clearly. Other single parents can also provide valuable support by enabling you to share disappointments and exchange advice with others who have faced similar challenges.

There are also community resources for single pregnant women; information can be found on the internet or at larger hospitals. Birth instructors and your hospital's women's centre or library often have information on smaller support groups that may suit you.

In a more mature couple, *conception can take much longer than in younger people and it is especially important that you give each other loving support.*

your career

Pregnancy and parenting will have significant effects on your life at work, your career progression, your work–life balance, and your finances. Therefore it pays to be aware of what to expect before becoming pregnant and to plan for your future as a working pregnant woman and a working mum.

THE PHYSICAL IMPACT OF PREGNANCY
No matter how fit you are, the physical changes of pregnancy will force you to slow down, especially in the first and third trimesters. For most women, the main pregnancy complaint is overwhelming tiredness. It can be frustrating to find you can no longer work for as many hours as before, or at the same intensity, especially if your career is very important to you. Also, as your pregnancy progresses, you will have to make time for increasingly frequent antenatal check-ups. So it's worth being prepared for the fact that things at work will need to slow down. However, for the most part, there is no reason why you can't continue to be effective in your work.

Complications during pregnancy, such as high blood pressure, are more common in

women over 35, as is Caesarean delivery. You may need to think about cutting down on your working hours earlier than younger women.

Your environment If you are exposed to chemicals that could harm your baby (see pp20–21), consider raising the subject of a planned pregnancy with your Human Resources manager to discuss the job changes that could take place once you are pregnant. If you don't want to discuss this with your employers, get advice from a colleague who has been pregnant.

CAREER PROGRESSION
Make sure you are aware of the demands parenting will make on you, and how these might impact on your work life. This way, you

Making realistic plans for pregnancy and parenthood will allow you to continue with your career successfully.

Maternity Leave and Pay

In the UK, women are entitled to up to 26 weeks leave from their employment, starting no earlier than 11 weeks before the expected week of childbirth. During this period, most women are entitled to statutory maternity pay (SMP). Some companies have more generous allowances than this, and it is worth contacting your Human Resources department or checking your terms and conditions of employment.

Statutory Maternity Pay This is paid by your employer for 26 weeks. If you qualify, SMP is paid for 6 weeks at 90 per cent of your average salary and for 20 weeks at a flat rate that is set by the government (in 2004, this was £102 a week). For women who do not qualify for SMP, Maternity Allowance is paid instead by the Benefits Agency. This is paid for 26 weeks at a rate of £102 a week.

Parental leave In addition to maternity leave (and paternity leave) parents are entitled to 13 weeks unpaid leave to be taken before the child is 5 years old. To qualify for parental leave you have to have been in your job for at least a year.

For more information on your rights, you can contact the Maternity Alliance or the Department of Trade and Industry (see pp154–155).

can be prepared for the challenges of juggling two very different parts of your life, with their clashing priorities. With good planning and a common-sense approach, there is no reason why your career cannot flourish while you become a parent. Look for role models who inspire you and help show you ways to carry off this complex juggling act. Examining the successes of women who went before you can help make the challenge seem more positive, while helping you to avoid pitfalls.

Family-friendly companies Some companies have liberal maternity leave policies, provide child care (either as a workplace nursery or money towards child-care costs), and will consider flexible work arrangements when you return to work. If you realize your employer does not have family-friendly policies, you (or your partner) may want to consider looking for other employment where more flexible working is possible. However, remember that extra maternity benefits often only apply once you have been working for a company for a certain period.

WORK–HOME BALANCE

Many women find that, when it comes to child care, they and their partners somehow revert to traditional roles, with the woman shouldering the bulk of the burden, despite the fact that they both work full-time. Therefore, it pays to assess as realistically as possible how a child will change your lives, and negotiate with your partner now about how you will share the responsibility.

Rethinking the balance Discuss the practicalities with your partner at this point, to establish your priorities and expectations of child care and parenthood, and how to fit family life with both of your careers. Perhaps this is the ideal opportunity for one of you to take a longed-for career break to look after the baby, or to work part-time and take on child care for the rest of the week. Perhaps one of you has a family-friendly employer who will offer that partner more flexibility to deal with child care responsibilities than the other's employer.

You may want to map out who will be responsible for what – the morning drop-offs to the nursery, the evening feeding and bathtime routines, and who will take time off work for your future child's postnatal check-ups or if your child becomes sick for a week. Thrashing out these things before the baby comes allows you both to know what to expect of the future and what is expected of yourselves. It will also allow you to plan how to get the most out of your working hours and feel in control of your career.

preconception medical care

Even if you consider yourself healthy, you may want to think about a visit to your doctor before you try to become pregnant. Such a visit can reassure you about any medications you are taking, and gives your doctor the opportunity to check for any preexisting medical conditions before you try to conceive. You can also make sure you are eating healthily and taking necessary supplements.

Often, the chief purpose of a check-up before conception is to reassure yourself that any medicines you take are safe in pregnancy or to change to more appropriate medications. In every case it is important to discuss with your doctor the effect that stopping the medication may have on your pregnancy compared with the effects that medication may have on a developing fetus. Many women stop taking prescribed drugs because of fears they may be harmful, when in fact they are vitally important to their health and therefore to the baby's health.

Another reason for a check-up is if there is any serious genetic disorder in your family or your partner's. In many cases you can be tested to see whether or not your baby is at risk.

Usually, the focus of any preconception visit is information gathering. Your doctor may ask

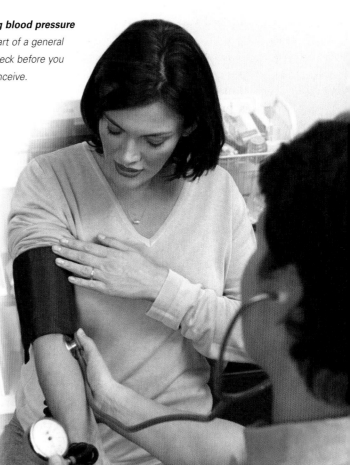

Checking blood pressure can be part of a general health check before you try to conceive.

Getting Informed

Not everyone needs a preconception check-up, but there are many benefits. You will get specific information about:

- How any medical conditions you have may affect your pregnancy.
- Whether you need to change any of the medications you taking.
- Whether your baby may be at risk of a genetic disorder, and in cases of genetic risk, what testing is available to you.
- Taking folic acid supplements (see p22), which protect against neural tube defects.

you an exhaustive list of questions or ask you to fill out a detailed health questionnaire.

ROUTINE CHECK-UPS

It's a good idea to get a basic physical examination with a general practitioner. At this visit, you can get your blood pressure checked, update any vaccinations you need, make sure you are not anaemic, and be screened for thyroid disorders. If your cervical smear is due you should have it done because options for evaluating an abnormal result while you are pregnant are very limited.

Immunity to diseases It's also a good idea to have a blood test to see if you are already immune to rubella (german measles). Contracting this disease during your pregnancy can be damaging to your baby. If you are not already immune, you can be immunized before pregnancy to protect both you and your baby. You should wait at least 3 months after immunizations before you try to become pregnant. Rubella in pregnancy can cause congenital problems such as deafness, cataracts, heart defects, and even death of the fetus.

Testing for infections You may also want to consider testing for certain infections that could affect your pregnancy or your baby. Testing for HIV and hepatitis B is usual before any form of assisted conception and is recommended

for all women wanting to become pregnant who are at risk (drug users and their partners). It is routine during early pregnancy in most antenatal clinics. Testing for other infections, such as herpes and hepatitis C, is not usually needed. Some doctors will check your immunity to toxoplasmosis (an infection that can be picked up when handling cat litter or through contact with garden soil). If you are not immune you should try to avoid dealing with cat litter or ensure you use gloves if there is no alternative.

GENETIC COUNSELLING

If anyone in your family or your partner's family has an inherited disease, such as Huntington's disease, you may be advised to see a genetic counsellor.

A counsellor will be able to advise you on the risks of your baby being affected by an inherited disease and what tests are available. Most couples will be offered amniocentesis or chorionic villus sampling (see pp58–59), but in some cases, couples may want to consider a new technique, which is called preimplantation genetic diagnosis in which the woman's eggs are fertilized by IVF and healthy embryos selected for implanting in the womb.

Genetic counselling is recommended for the following:
- Ashkenazi Jews, who have a higher risk of Tay–Sachs disease, Canavan disease, cystic fibrosis and other diseases.

- African Americans, who are at risk of sickle cell anaemia.
- Couples of Mediterranean descent, who are at a higher risk of the blood disorder beta-thalassaemia.
- Southeast Asians, who are at a higher risk of blood disorders such as alpha-thalassaemia.

DIET AND NUTRITION

It is important that you eat healthily if you are trying to conceive (see pp22–23). You need to take folic acid supplements (400mcg/day) to reduce the risk of neural tube defects in your baby (see p22). If you have a weight problem, you should address this before you become pregnant.

High–risk Disorders

Certain medical conditions can influence your chances of conceiving or present risks to your health, or that of your baby. If you have any of the following conditions you should see your doctor before you try to conceive. See p18–19 for more information.

- Diabetes
- Thyroid disorders
- Systemic lupus erythematosus
- High blood pressure
- Epilepsy
- Asthma
- Anaemia
- Hepatitis C or HIV infection
- Obesity, underweight, or eating disorders

preexisting medical conditions

At your preconception check you will need to discuss any medical conditions you may have, some of which can affect your ability to conceive, or which may in themselves be affected by pregnancy. Some conditions will need extra monitoring and you may need to switch medications.

DIABETES

If you have diabetes you will need special care before and during pregnancy to be sure that your blood sugar is well-controlled. The goals for your blood sugar values are less than 5mmol/l for your fasting blood sugar and less than 7.8mmol/l 2 hours after meals. As long as you are rigorous about this, you have a very good chance of having a healthy pregnancy and a healthy baby. If you have long-standing diabetes, you are more likely to develop certain pregnancy complications, especially preeclampsia (see p113). Any eye problems related to the diabetes may also worsen. High blood sugar levels at the time of conception can damage the developing baby so it is important to control blood sugar before you try to conceive – miscarriage is more likely, as are major birth defects such as neural tube defects or congenital heart disease. High blood sugar during pregnancy slows fetal lung development so the baby may have breathing problems at birth.

During your pregnancy it is important that you are screened early for neural tube defects, with a blood test or an ultrasound scan. If you are taking pills for diabetes, it is usually best if you switch to insulin before conception because it doesn't cross into the placenta. It is essential to continue to control your blood sugar. A first trimester evaluation of your vision and of your kidney function is also important. From 28 weeks your obstetrician may arrange extra scans to check fetal growth and well-being. These are usually every 4 weeks but may be more frequent.

SYSTEMIC LUPUS ERYTHEMATOSUS (SLE)

Women with this disorder can have healthy pregnancies, but it is best if conception happens when the condition is controlled. Most SLE medications are safe during pregnancy – active SLE is much more dangerous to your baby than the drugs used for treatment.

There is an increased risk of miscarriage or of the baby being small. About 1 in 80 babies will be born with heart problems. Your blood will be checked for signs of anti-phospholipid antibody syndrome. This condition increases the risk of blood clots developing as well as causing problems with the baby. If you have anti-phospholipid antibody syndrome, you will be treated with blood thinning injections during pregnancy to prevent a blood clot.

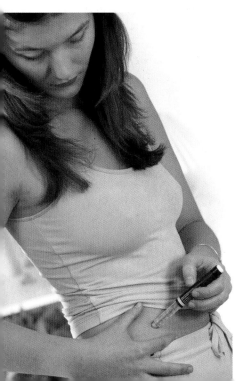

Insulin injections are safe during pregnancy and play an important part in controlling blood sugar levels in diabetes.

Your doctor is likely to start extra monitoring at around 32 weeks to check your baby's well-being. You will also have ultrasound scans to check the baby's growth and labour may be induced early.

EPILEPSY

Most anti-epileptic agents are linked with an increased risk of birth defects. To minimize this risk, consultation with your neurologist is needed to reduce the number of medications you are taking and the dose to the lowest levels possible that still control your fits, although changes in medication may affect you being able to drive. If you are taking anti-seizure medications, you should have screening for neural tube defects at 15 weeks and a detailed ultrasound between 20 and 22 weeks.

HYPOTHYROIDISM

Your body's need for thyroid hormone rises dramatically during the first half of pregnancy. This increased need may begin as early as 1 week after your missed period. As soon as you know you are pregnant you should see your doctor and get your thyroid function checked. In the US, women are recommended to increase their levothyroxine dose by one-third straight away.

Your thyroid function will probably be checked 3–4 times during your pregnancy and your medication adjusted as necessary. Treatment of hypothyroidism in pregnancy is very important; even borderline low thyroid hormone levels may affect your baby's brain and nervous system development. Screening for thyroid function is recommended in women over 35 with any autoimmune condition such as SLE or diabetes, or in women with a strong family history of thyroid disease.

OBESITY

If you are obese (body mass index over 30) you are more likely to develop problems in pregnancy (including miscarriage), some of which may be due to unrecognized diabetes. You are also more likely to develop diabetes and high blood pressure. Obese women often need a Caesarean delivery and have a higher rate of complications.

HIGH BLOOD PRESSURE

If you are being treated for high blood pressure you should see a doctor before conceiving. Some drugs used to treat high blood pressure should be avoided – your doctor will make sure you take a type that is safe. You may be at risk of complications such as preeclampsia (see p113) during your pregnancy. It is important that your kidney function is checked in the first trimester so that if protein is found in your urine later in the pregnancy you have a point of reference. Your doctor may suggest increased monitoring of your baby later in the pregnancy. It is vital that you take your medication during pregnancy – high blood pressure can cause bleeding in the placenta and be harmful to the baby.

DEPRESSION

Depression may worsen with the stresses of pregnancy and the accompanying hormonal shifts that take place. For this reason, you should not abruptly stop your antidepressant medication without medical supervision. Serotonin reuptake inhibitors (SSRIs) such as fluoxetine and sertraline can be continued during pregnancy.

Your doctor should communicate closely with your mental health provider before making any changes in medications.

ACNE

Acne can worsen in pregnancy. Before you conceive, ask your doctor about the safety of your current treatments. Isotretinoin can cause significant birth defects, and any woman taking this drug should be using a reliable form of birth control. Do not take any antibiotics for acne without checking with your obstetrician.

environmental hazards

Anything that you expose your body to, whether it is foods you eat or pollutants such as cigarette smoke, can affect your body and, potentially, your unborn baby. It is therefore especially important before conception and around the time of conception to be aware how things in your everyday life may affect your chances of becoming pregnant and the health of your baby.

In many cases, scientists have not adequately studied the effects of environmental factors on human fertility. One of the reasons is that often it is difficult to isolate one risk factor, such as pesticide exposure, from other risk factors for lower fertility. However, it is sensible to avoid certain known hazards.

FOOD AND ALCOHOL

Some foods are potentially hazardous mainly because they may be contaminated with pollutants (such as mercury) or microorganisms (such as listeriosis) that cause disease. These are covered more fully on pages 48–49. Coffee and alcohol intake may also influence fertility.

Coffee Drinking coffee is unlikely to reduce your chances of conceiving unless you drink a lot. More than five cups a day may slightly lower your fertility. Try to limit your overall caffeine intake to 250–300mg. An "average" cup of coffee has about 90mg of caffeine. Remember that tea and certain soft drinks often contain caffeine.

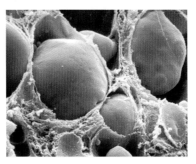

Egg development *may be hindered by toxins such as cigarette smoke. This highly magnified image shows eggs maturing in the ovary.*

Alcohol This is linked with some reduction in fertility, but only if you drink more than 4–8 alcoholic beverages a week. An occasional drink is unlikely to significantly affect your ability to conceive. However, it is best to refrain from binge drinking, mainly so that you don't have to worry about the possible effects on your baby if you do become pregnant.

SMOKING

Smoking causes significant decreases in fertility. It's estimated that about 13 per cent of cases of infertility may be attributable to cigarette smoking. Smoking also reduces the amount of oxygen reaching your baby.

Smoking also lowers the age at which women start menopause, suggesting that it contributes to the premature depletion of eggs in the ovaries. Unfortunately, infertility in smokers cannot always be treated successfully with assisted reproductive technology (ART) because smoking can permanently affect the ability of your ovaries to respond to fertility treatments. Smoking marijuana has also been linked to decreased fertility, especially when it is combined with alcohol.

The best time to stop smoking is now, before you become pregnant.

this is an **ideal time** to assess environmental **hazards** in your life

X-RAYS AND RADIATION

The amount of radiation in routine X-rays should not affect your ability to become pregnant in the future. However, women who have had pelvic radiation for cancer are likely to have problems conceiving. The level of radiation in any one diagnostic X-ray should not increase your risk of miscarriage; however, it is always a good idea to tell the technician if you are trying to conceive so that your uterus can be shielded.

INFECTIONS

Some infections can increase your chance of miscarriage, but most common infections, such as influenza and the common cold, do not. Chickenpox (varicella) and rubella are potential problems if contracted around conception or during pregnancy. If you are unsure whether you have had either of these infections, ask your doctor to check if you are immune. If necessary, you can get vaccinated before conceiving. Rubella vaccine should not be given if you are already pregnant or trying to conceive.

Most women over 35 are already immune to parvovirus and toxoplasmosis. No vaccination is available, and testing prior to pregnancy is not recommended. While trying to conceive (and during pregnancy) you can reduce the risk of toxoplasmosis by asking your partner to clean the cat litter tray and by washing your hands carefully after handling raw meat.

WHAT'S SAFE AND WHAT'S NOT?

■ **Are pesticides a risk to my unborn baby?**

Few studies have systematically studied the relationship between fertility and pesticide exposure at home. However, it probably makes sense to purchase organically grown produce and to wash carefully all fruits and vegetables while you are trying to become pregnant. Limit the use of pesticides and herbicides that you handle in your garden.

■ **Is passive smoking dangerous to my baby?**

While secondhand smoke is a health hazard to you over time, the effects of occasional secondhand smoke on your fertility and pregnancy are likely to be fairly small. It makes sense to avoid enclosed areas with intense levels of secondhand smoke such as bars and pubs, and to discourage others from smoking in your home. In addition, strong smells such as that from smoke may worsen the symptoms of nausea and vomiting during pregnancy.

■ **What about the risk of mercury poisoning?**

Higher mercury levels have been linked with decreased fertility and can also cause problems in the developing baby. Much of our mercury intake comes from eating certain fish. The UK Food Standards Agency advise that women who are pregnant or trying to conceive should avoid eating shark, marlon, and swordfish because they may contain high levels of mercury. You should also limit the amount of tuna you eat. Don't eat more than four medium-sized tins of tuna or two fresh tuna steaks per week. Mercury can stay in your system for a long time, so be careful with your fish intake 6 months before becoming pregnant.

■ **Should I avoid microwaves and computers?**

No studies so far have found a convincing link to either low fertility rates or miscarriage. The amount of radiation released by these devices is very small – less than many natural sources, such as solar radiation. Microwaves cannot penetrate your skin more than a fraction of an inch.

■ **Is it safe to use hair dye?**

Very little hair dye is absorbed through your skin when you colour your hair and should pose no risk to your fertility.

■ **What other chemicals should be avoided?**

Strong-smelling chemicals, such as paints, solvents, and cleaning products, are best avoided while you are pregnant or trying to conceive. If you cannot avoid strong-smelling chemicals, make sure you wear gloves, a mask, and protective clothing. Always work in a well-ventilated area.

nutrition and exercise

Good nutrition and targeted exercise during the months prior to conception can improve your physical and emotional health. For mature parents-to-be, replenishing your resources for conception and pregnancy can make it easier to conceive and can help you have an easier labour and birth.

Folic Acid

Folic acid is an important nutrient around the time of conception. Although it is found naturally in several foods, it is recommended women take a supplement to make sure they have an adequate intake of this important vitamin.

Folic acid decreases the risk of neural tube birth defects, which affect the brain and spinal cord. Neural tube defects occur during the first 28 days after conception, which is before most women realize they are pregnant. Making sure that you have enough folic acid before conception can reduce the risk of neural tube defects by as much as 70 per cent.

- You should ideally start taking folic acid supplements at least 3 months before you conceive.
- The recommended intake is 0.4mg every day.
- Aim also to include two portions of fruit and vegetables that are rich in folic acid, such as papaya and asparagus. Most breads, grains, and breakfast cereals are also enriched with folic acid.

Being in the best of health and fitness will allow you as much control over pregnancy and birth as possible. The best time to get into shape is before pregnancy, so a sensible diet and regular fitness will allow you to reap the rewards later.

EATING WELL

Healthy eating will have a very positive impact on your general health and your hormonal balance and give your body the best chance to conceive. Eating a good variety of freshly prepared, well-balanced meals will give you all the nutrients you need. Try to include all the main food groups – meat and fish, cereal and grains, fruit and vegetables and dairy foods – and reduce your intake of processed foods, ready meals, and refined sugars. Select unsaturated fats over saturated ones and eat carbohydrates regularly but in moderation. Choose complex

Eat a variety of fresh fruits and vegetables – seven portions a day is recommended. If you can, choose organic produce. Fruit juice counts as one portion of fruit.

carbohydrates (such as whole grains, legumes, vegetables, and fruits) over simple or fast-releasing carbohydrates (such as refined white flour and sugar, which give you plenty of calories but less of the nutrients).

Fibre is vital to a healthy diet, and a regular intake of protein is a must. Also, do not underestimate the importance of water – aim to drink at least six glasses a day.

YOUR BODYWEIGHT

Your pre-pregnancy weight affects your well-being during pregnancy and your baby's birthweight.

Being very overweight decreases fertility in both men and women. In addition, obese women are more likely to miscarry and to experience complications in pregnancy, such as gestational diabetes and high blood pressure. They are also more likely to encounter problems during birth.

Being underweight can also be a problem. Women who are underweight often do not ovulate regularly, which decreases their chances of conception. They are more likely to give birth to underweight babies. It's best to take corrective action before you conceive – your health will improve and your pregnancy is likely to be less complicated.

FITNESS PLAN

The list of benefits of exercise before and after you conceive is long. Good overall physical health, weight control, a positive body

---

Can You Exercise Too Much?

Moderate exercise will not decrease your chances of conceiving or put you at risk for miscarriage. However, competitive women athletes tend to ovulate irregularly or not at all. Therefore, if you exercise at a very high intensity and for several hours a day, you may want to pay special attention to assessing your ovulation each month (see p24). If you find that you are ovulating, athletic training will not lower your chances to conceive.

---

image, emotional balance, and stress reduction top the list for couples who are trying to conceive. Fit women also have lower rates of some of the complications during pregnancy that are more common in older mums, such as high blood pressure and diabetes, and can expect easier labours and recoveries after the birth of their babies.

Beginning an exercise programme The intense fatigue right at the start of your pregnancy makes beginning an exercise programme at that point much more difficult than it is before. Therefore, the optimal time to set up an exercise programme is right now. If you are obese or are diabetic, consult your health care provider first.

The ideal exercise programme includes an aerobic activity, some strength training, and flexibility exercises. All three together build great overall health.

Aerobic activities Exercise such as walking, swimming, and cycling improves the efficiency of your lungs, heart, and circulatory system. It also helps enhance your

emotional well-being, and promote more restful sleep.

To be effective, aerobic exercise has to last at least 30 minutes and raise your heart rate adequately. The easiest way to know that you have reached your optimal heart rate is to keep track of how out of breath you are during your activity. If you still can just maintain a conversation with an exercise partner throughout your activity, you are exercising at the correct intensity for your body. You can also use a heart-rate monitor to check your heart rate.

Strength training Activities such as weight training and Pilates build muscle strength. Abdominal muscle strength helps protect you from back pain during pregnancy, as well as for the rest of your life.

Flexibility Stretching prevents injuries by relaxing your muscles and increasing your range of motion. It also decreases soreness and contributes to your sense of well-being by promoting deep breathing, relaxation, and good blood flow. Yoga and dance moves are both good for flexibility.

understanding your fertility

Age has a clear influence on fertility. A woman's fertility starts to decline after the age of 35, as a result of a number of factors including a decrease in the number and health of her eggs, an increasing likelihood of medical problems such as diabetes, and less frequent intercourse. By understanding your fertility it is possible to optimize your chances of conception.

Statistics make assumptions about your health and lifestyle that may not apply to your individual situation. Therefore, while you will have to allow for the possibility of a longer conception time, it is best to assume that you will become pregnant within a year or so, and confidently make plans to achieve conception.

Most couples conceive within one year of unprotected sex. However, couples using timed intercourse can conceive twice as fast. Timed intercourse involves finding the most fertile days in your cycle and then having sex around this time.

PREDICTING OVULATION

There are several methods to determine your fertile days (or your time of ovulation). It is best to find the one that you like best and then use it consistently.

Rhythm method and ovulation calculators Both these methods determine your fertile period using the interval between

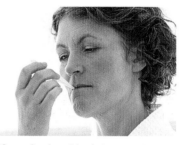

Measuring basal body temperature (BBT) throughout your cycle can help predict the day you are likely to ovulate. A BBT thermometer can detect very small changes in temperature.

menstrual periods (usually 28–30 days). To find your fertile window, subtract 14 days from your cycle length (for example, if your cycle is 30 days from the start of one menstrual period to the next, subtract 14 from 30, giving 16). This number is your estimated day of ovulation and you are most likely to be fertile.

Ovulation counters work on exactly the same principle but they do the maths for you. The rhythm method is unreliable for cycle lengths shorter than 21 days or longer than 35 days, but is imperfect even in women with regular 28-day cycles.

Optimizing Intercourse for Conception

There are several ways to increase your chances of conception by varying when and how you have intercourse.

■ **Frequency** Advice on how often to have intercourse varies. Some experts suggest having sex on four of the six most fertile days, others recommend sex every second or third day. However, daily or infrequent (less than every 10–14 days) intercourse is probably detrimental to sperm count.

■ **Sexual position** Some experts recommend that the woman remain lying down for 20 minutes after intercourse to minimize leakage of sperm from the vagina, but there's no evidence it improves conception.

■ **Sexual enjoyment** Women who climax when having sex appear to conceive faster – orgasm causes vaginal and uterine movements that encourage the movement of sperm into the uterus and fallopian tubes.

Basal body temperature Your resting body temperature (basal body temperature or BBT) rises by about 0.3°C (0.5°F) right after ovulation. This temperature change can be checked accurately with a BBT thermometer, which can measure very small changes in temperature. BBT should be taken every morning at the same time before you get up. Record it for 3 or 4 months so you can see your ovulation pattern and use it to predict subsequent ovulations.

Cervical mucus The consistency and colour of cervical mucus changes throughout your monthly cycle (see right). As you approach the middle of your cycle, your mucus will change from its usual opaque and sticky feel. During the days when you are most fertile, your mucus will be clear, slippery, and stretchy. To test your cervical mucus, collect some secretions from your vagina with your index finger. If the mucus is clear and forms a thin filament between your finger and your thumb, you are at your most fertile.

Ovulation prediction kits These tests detect the rise in luteinizing hormone (LH) 2–3 days before ovulation. You need to calculate the days you are most likely to be fertile, then test for LH every day for several days before and after. Each test provides you with a positive or negative result for each given day only. The kits are expensive and not always reliable.

Changes During the Menstrual Cycle

The menstrual cycle is a result of a complex interaction of hormones. Rising levels of follicle stimulating hormone (FSH) encourage eggs to mature in follicles within the ovaries. This also promotes the production of oestrogen. A surge in luteinizing hormone (LH) triggers the mature egg to be released, simultaneously triggering a rise in body temperature. In the second half of the cycle (after ovulation), progesterone (produced by the burst egg follicle) halts FSH and LH production and continues the thickening of the womb lining so that it is ready to receive a fertilized egg. Cervical secretions change throughout the cycle.

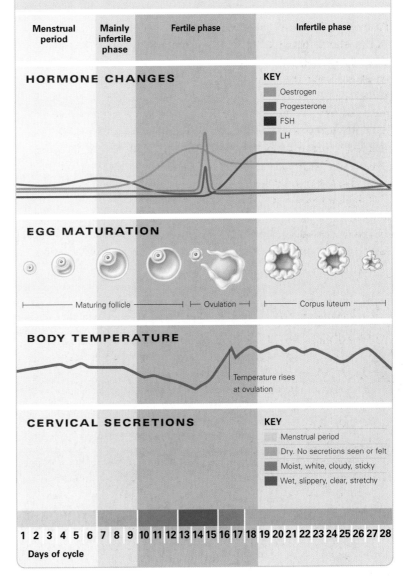

problems conceiving

It's perfectly normal for it to take longer to conceive as you get older, but rather than wait too long for nature to take its course, it's worth seeking medical advice if you haven't conceived within 6 months of trying, although it may take 12 months before you are referred to a gynaecologist.

It is a fact that fertility decreases with age, and women who wait until they are over 35 to have children are more likely to have problems conceiving than their younger counterparts. However, being over 35 does not mean that you will not be able to become pregnant, but in most cases it does take longer. The decrease in fertility as women get older is probably due to several factors. First, there is a greater risk of unrecognized miscarriage as a result of chromosomal problems. Late or irregular menstrual cycles may actually represent very early miscarriage. Second, aging may affect the uterus. For example, older women are more likely to have fibroids (a growth of fibrous tissue in the uterus), which may lower the chances of a fertilized egg implanting successfully.

PLANNING FOR SUCCESS

Even if you haven't conceived yet, you probably still can. Only 1 per cent of all couples are considered sterile, which means they will never be able to become pregnant. If you have been trying for a few months you might want to reassess lifestyle factors and ovulation prediction, but don't wait too long before seeking help.

Re-check your ovulation prediction Targeted intercourse raises your chance of conception significantly. However, success is likely only if you correctly predict your fertile days (see pp24–25).

Maintain a healthy lifestyle Lifestyle choices probably have only small effects on your fertility. However, if you are having problems conceiving you will want to maximize your chances by eliminating anything that may have a detrimental effect. Check your caffeine and alcohol intake

---

Understanding Conception

When a mature egg is released from the ovaries it is carried along the fallopian tube towards the uterus. Fertilization usually occurs in the fallopian tube, with one of many competing sperm penetrating the egg. At this point, the nucleus (central part) of the sperm fuses with the egg's nucleus. The fertilized egg divides first to become two cells, then four, eight and so on. The fertilized egg embeds in the uterus 5–7 days after fertilization.

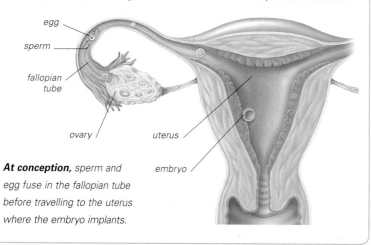

egg
sperm
fallopian tube
ovary
uterus
embryo

At conception, sperm and egg fuse in the fallopian tube before travelling to the uterus where the embryo implants.

to make sure you are minimizing your exposure. To preserve your sanity even more than to boost your fertility, you should take measures to reduce your stress levels. Keeping up a regular exercise programme will help. Boost your general well-being by eating a healthy diet (see pp22–23). It's all too easy to start off with great intentions and then revert to old patterns. Try to invigorate your daily commitment to a healthy lifestyle by focusing on changes you can make with the least amount of effort and those you can make together as a couple.

WHEN TO SEEK HELP

GPs take the age of parents-to-be very seriously and while a waiting time of up to 1 year is reasonable for women under 30, most doctors will begin testing and treating women over 35 after 6 months of trying to become pregnant. Women over 40 are able to receive fertility testing right from the start. This is because the chances of conceiving naturally decline fairly steadily after 35. By age 40, around one-third of couples are likely to have problems becoming pregnant. After age 40, two-thirds of women have fertility problems.

You can also get help from natural family planning and infertility support groups (see pp154–155) who can provide advice, resources, and open minds. Gathering information about infertility treatments may also make you feel more in control of

the conception process. Often, more specific knowledge about available treatments can put you more at ease and reduce your anxiety.

If you do decide to consult with a fertility specialist, make sure you ask to be referred to one who listens carefully and offers you a range of options.

Many doctors recommend psychological counselling for couples with infertility issues, especially if IVF is likely to be an option. If the monthly rollercoaster of hope and disappointment has resulted in serious frustration or if planned

sex has zapped your relationship, you may want to consider seeing a counsellor, even without medical infertility intervention.

BEGINNING TREATMENT

Depending on your age and health, you might decide that you need to see an infertility specialist quickly. Various health conditions, such as irregular menstrual periods, may make this advisable (see above). Consider the impact various treatments may have on your daily schedule, your finances, and your emotional well-being.

HEALTH QUESTIONNAIRE

■ **Do you have problems with your menstrual periods?**
If your menstrual periods are irregular or unpredictable, you may need to have tests to determine if you are ovulating regularly. If you have heavy or painful periods you should be evaluated for endometriosis, which can affect fertility. In this condition, tissue that lines the uterus lodges in other parts of the pelvic area, including the fallopian tubes and ovaries.

■ **Have you ever been told you have had pelvic inflammatory disease (PID)?**
PID can cause scarring of the fallopian tubes, which may then become blocked. If you are having fertility problems, your tubes should be checked by tests (see p28). If they are blocked you may need IVF.

■ **Have you or your partner ever completed cancer treatment?**
Some cancer treatments, especially radiation treatment, can affect sperm and egg production. In some cases, eggs or sperm can be collected before any treatment if there is a risk of infertility, and used later in assisted conception.

■ **Are you concerned you may not be ovulating?**
A medical check-up is appropriate if, for example, your basal body temperature or your cervical mucus do not change throughout your cycle.

■ **Have you ever had more than two miscarriages?**
Doctors usually recommend chromosome analysis in you and your partner as well as other tests.

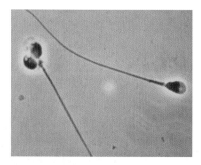

Abnormal sperm, such as the double-headed sperm on the left of this highly magnified sample, is a possible cause of infertility in men.

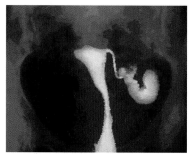

A blocked fallopian tube can cause fertility problems. Dye passed through the cervix flows into the narrow tube on the right, but the left tube is blocked.

TESTS AND INVESTIGATIONS

The infertility evaluation begins with tests to make sure that your partner has normal sperm, you are ovulating, and that your fallopian tubes are open. Almost one half of infertility problems are caused by problems with sperm production. Evaluation of male factor infertility relies on testing a sample of sperm from your partner. Sperm may be abnormal in shape, or your partner may have low sperm numbers. To confirm that you are ovulating, your doctor will ask for detailed information about your menstrual cycles; one of the best signs of ovulation is regular and predictable menstrual cycles, but your doctor will also arrange blood tests to check your hormone levels. One of the most informative tests is based on levels of follicle-stimulating hormone (FSH) on the third day after your menstrual cycle begins. FSH stimulates the ovaries, so your body's need for high levels early in your cycle may indicate that your ovaries have less reserve than normal or that the quality of your eggs is reduced.

If your partner's sperm is normal and you are ovulating normally, your doctor will need to look for other explanations. Your gynaecologist may perform a test called a hysterosalpingogram to evaluate the inside of your uterus and to see if your fallopian tubes are open. Dye is placed into your uterus using a small tube that is placed through your cervix. This dye travels up into the tubes, revealing any blockage or problems with your uterus.

Other possible tests may include a hysteroscopy (where a telescope is placed through your cervix to examine the inside of your uterus) or a laparoscopy (where a telescope is surgically placed into your abdomen to examine your uterus, ovaries, and tubes from the outside).

Once your evaluation is complete, your doctor will review the results with you and your partner. If the tests reveal your ovaries are unable to produce eggs, donor eggs are a potential option (see p31). In about 15 per cent of cases, no explanation will be found for why you are having trouble conceiving, but unexplained infertility still responds to fertility treatments.

Choosing a Fertility Specialist

Many fertility centres try to impress you with their success rates, but other factors are just as important.

■ Find a gynaecologist who has experience in infertility.

■ If choosing a clinic with a high success rate is important to you, be careful to compare like with like. Try to obtain pregnancy success rates for women your age, and ask about the practice's rate of twins and triplets. Clinics carrying out more treatment cycles have higher success rates. But you don't have to go to the busiest clinic: above 138 cycles a year, rates doesn't improve with more women treated..

■ Make sure you are comfortable with your doctor, and the nursing and office staff. Infertility treatment is a stressful time; being treated with respect and feeling comfortable about obtaining information and having all your questions answered eases the process.

assisted conception

Medical advances are allowing more women to have children – even those who have tried to conceive for many years. Since fertility problems are much more common as you get older, women over 35 are prime candidates for assisted conception.

The hallmark of assisted reproduction (ART) is ovulation induction. Stimulation of your ovaries can be done alone, or in combination with assisted fertilization. In women with polycystic ovary disease (PCO), treatment with fertility pills (clomiphene citrate) with or without a medication called metformin may be enough to help you become pregnant.

In women who do not respond to pills alone, the next step is a combination of hormone injections (gonadotropins) and assisted fertilization. Your partner can usually administer these injections at home. During your hormone treatment, the clinic will carefully monitor egg production by your ovaries with frequent ultrasound scans. If your ovaries respond well, you will be given human chorionic gonadotropin (hCG), which triggers ovulation. At the same time, your doctor will introduce a sample of your partner's sperm into your uterus – a procedure known as intrauterine insemination (IUI.)

If your fallopian tubes are blocked, your partner's sperm

count is very low, or other treatments have failed, you will probably be offered in vitro fertilization (IVF). With this technique, the same hormone treatments are used to stimulate your ovaries, but instead of IUI, your eggs are collected from your ovaries through a needle guided by ultrasound (see p30). In standard IVF, your eggs are then combined with your partner's sperm in a Petri dish in the laboratory.

Sperm meets egg in this specialized type of IVF called ISCI, where an individual sperm is injected directly into the egg.

If your difficulties conceiving are due to problems with your partner's sperm, microscopic techniques are used to inject a single sperm into each of your eggs, a procedure known as intra-cytoplasmic sperm injection (ICSI).

After fertilization, healthy embryos are returned to your

uterus using a narrow tube (catheter) placed through your cervix. After the embryos are transferred, you will be checked regularly for signs of a successful pregnancy. This is done using a combination of blood testing and ultrasound scans.

Each combination of hormonal stimulation, egg retrieval, fertilization, and embryo transfer is referred to as an IVF cycle.

TREATMENT SIDE EFFECTS

Treatment with hormones is no picnic. On top of having to give yourself an injection every day, the combination of hormones and the stress of worrying about whether the treatment will work is likely to make you moody and irritable. On top of this, your ovaries will enlarge considerably leaving you feeling bloated and sometimes causing abdominal discomfort. In certain cases, the ovaries are overstimulated by the hormone treatment and the IVF cycle may need to be cancelled – in other words, doctors will not proceed to the egg retrieval stage. The cycle could also be cancelled if your ovaries do not respond to hormone treatments. This is more likely in women over the age of 35.

SUCCESS RATES

Your chance of pregnancy with ART will depend on several factors. Often, the doctor will not know what your individual chances are until he or she can evaluate how well your body responds to hormonal stimulation. To get the best idea, ask what the success rates are for women your age. In the US, success rates per IVF cycle are 27 per cent for women aged 35–37, 18.5 per cent for women aged 38–40, and 7.3 per cent in women over 40. Success rates vary hugely in the UK.

POTENTIAL RISKS

The main risk of ART is that you will become pregnant with twins, triplets, quadruplets, or even more. The more babies you carry, the greater the chances of developing complications in pregnancy. This is especially true with triplets or more. The most serious complication with a multiple pregnancy is an increased risk of miscarriage or very early preterm labour (less than 28 weeks of pregnancy), which can result in more than one very sick baby who could have long-term

In Vitro Fertilization (IVF) Explained

In IVF, hormone treatments are used to stimulate your ovaries to produce eggs, which are then collected from your ovaries through a narrow flexible tube guided by ultrasound. Depending on the success of hormone stimulation, up to 10 or 12 eggs may be collected. Your eggs are then either combined with your partner's sperm in a dish in the laboratory or injected with a single sperm into each of your eggs, a procedure known as intracytoplasmic sperm injection (ICSI). After fertilization, healthy embryos are selected and returned to your uterus through a narrow tube (catheter) placed through your vagina and cervix. The tube is then slowly removed.

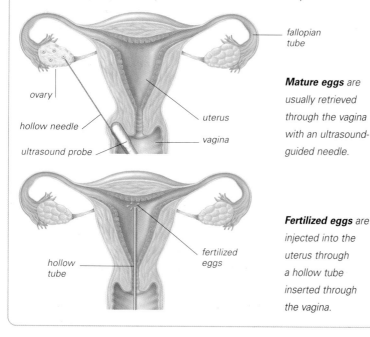

ovary

hollow needle

ultrasound probe

fallopian tube

uterus

vagina

Mature eggs are usually retrieved through the vagina with an ultrasound-guided needle.

hollow tube

fertilized eggs

Fertilized eggs are injected into the uterus through a hollow tube inserted through the vagina.

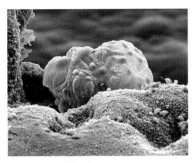

A newly fertilized egg starts to embed in the lining of the uterus.

DONATED EGGS

■ **Why might the doctor recommend using donor eggs?**

Donor eggs are not widely available in the UK, and demand is very much greater than supply. There are several reasons why donor eggs may be recommended: you may have had an early menopause or do not ovulate; there may be a risk of serious inherited disease; tests may have found you have poor eggs.

■ **How are donor eggs selected?**

You can choose anonymous egg donation, where you choose a donor based on age, ethnic background, and education, or you can ask a family member or friend to donate for you.

■ **How does this differ from IVF?**

Donor eggs are fertilized with your partner's sperm and then placed inside your uterus in a process similar to IVF.

■ **What are the costs and legal implications?**

In general, you should not need to worry about legal concerns since donors waive their parental rights as part of the process. Using donor eggs is usually very costly and this technology is unlikely to be available on the NHS.

■ **What are the advantages of using donor eggs?**

Using donor eggs reduces the risk that your baby will have a chromosomal abnormality (egg donors are usually under 30). If you are over 40, using donor eggs substantially increases the chance that you will become pregnant. Although the child is not genetically related to you, you will experience every other aspect of pregnancy, including the delivery. However, some women find having a baby that is genetically unrelated to them is psychologically difficult.

health problems. It is important that you discuss these risks with your fertility specialist up front. Triplets may result from treatment with clomiphene citrate alone, but if you are having IVF you may want to talk candidly with your doctor about the risks and benefits. Many specialists limit the number of embryos transferred to 2 to reduce the chances of pregnancy with triplets or more.

Many women also worry about the risk of having a baby with a birth defect due to IVF. Up to 4 per cent of babies conceived naturally are born with some form of birth defect. In women who have undergone IVF, the risk is higher – 9 per cent in one study. However, this increased risk may not be due to the IVF, but rather to the fact that couples receiving infertility treatment are already more likely to have problems with their eggs or sperm. The good news is that 91–95 per cent of babies born after IVF are healthy.

At one point, there was concern that repeatedly stimulating the ovaries with hormones may increase the risks of subsequent ovarian cancer. However, more recent research has shown that while ovarian cancer is more common in women with infertility, IVF may not further increase your risks.

CHECKING OUT THE COST

IVF is expensive and most medical insurance will not cover it. Most regions of the UK will offer some free IVF, but the number of cycles is strictly controlled as are the couples who are referred. Most areas limit NHS IVF treatment by the age of the woman and to those who do not already have children. The clinics are accustomed to questions about financial aspects of IVF, so don't be embarrassed about getting information on the exact costs of each step in your evaluation and treatment.

miscarriage

Many women worry about the risk of miscarriage, and it is common – about 10–20 per cent of recognized pregnancies end in miscarriage. However, although the risk is greater the older you are, most women over 35 will have completely normal pregnancies. Most miscarriages happen in the first 12 weeks of pregnancy; after this stage you can start to relax.

Vaginal bleeding is a common sign of miscarriage, but miscarriage can occur without any symptoms. Conversely, just because you have some bleeding, do not panic. Call your doctor but remember that in half of all cases of first trimester bleeding the pregnancy continues normally. Symptoms such as breast tenderness or nausea are generally good signs that the pregnancy is fine.

Once your doctor has been able to detect a normal heartbeat, the chances of a miscarriage are low, even if you are having a little bit of bleeding. A fetal heart rate of more than 100 beats per minute at 6 weeks gestation is an especially good sign. If you have first trimester screening for Down syndrome and have normal results, the chances of miscarriage are even less.

CAUSES OF MISCARRIAGE

The most important fact to realize about miscarriage is that most pregnancies that end in miscarriage were not normal. Early miscarriage is generally a sign that a genetic or developmental problem happened very early during your pregnancy. It is not your fault. You did not cause your miscarriage by drinking a glass of wine, dancing the night away, running up a flight of stairs, making love with your partner, working at a

Coping with miscarriage is particularly difficult. A supportive partner can help you come to terms with your loss.

computer screen, or almost anything else you can think of. Even direct trauma to your abdomen, as might occur with a car accident, is unlikely to hurt your baby early in pregnancy because the uterus is protected by the bony pelvis.

Genetic abnormalities These are the most common cause of miscarriage and are usually present from the moment of conception. Since genetic glitches are

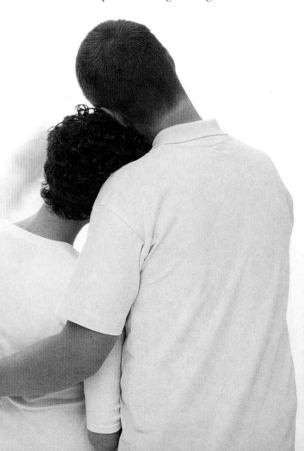

Recurrent Miscarriage

Since miscarriage is so common, a single miscarriage doesn't make doctors concerned that another miscarriage is likely. If you have had a single miscarriage in the past, try not to let anxiety consume you; the odds are in your favour that you can expect a completely normal pregnancy this time. If you have had two miscarriages or more, it is still very likely that you are completely normal. However, after three miscarriages, most experts recommend that you see a gynaecologist to make sure there is no treatable reason for your pregnancy losses.

more common as women get older, miscarriage due to this problem is directly related to your age. However, the risk of miscarriage in women over 35 is still only slightly higher than in younger women.

Developmental abnormalities Normal development is a very complicated process. In some cases, miscarriage results from a "wrong turn" in this process and is more common in women with uncontrolled diabetes or those taking certain drugs.

Maternal factors Polycystic ovarian syndrome and obesity are both associated with an increased risk.

Cervical incompetence In this condition, also referred to as cervical insufficiency, the cervix (the opening to the uterus) opens up before it should. The condition is not common, but it can cause pregnancy loss later in pregnancy (see p111).

EMOTIONAL RECOVERY

The abrupt and unwanted end of your pregnancy can be a tremendous loss, especially if you had tried to conceive for many months and were aware of your baby before your miscarriage. Although your pain may not always be recognized by some people, it is important to acknowledge it yourself and to take effective steps to heal before trying to conceive again. Many people may feel uncomfortable about talking to you about a miscarriage – they may make comments that are intended to make you feel better, but that are unintentionally offensive. Try not to get angry; people may find it difficult to understand what this loss means to you.

Take time to mourn your loss Grieving is an individual process, and everyone handles grief in his or her own way. However, there are recognized stages that you may go through. Often, grieving begins with avoidance – this allows you to manage your life despite the intense pain you may feel. Then, when you are ready to deal with your loss, you allow yourself to feel your pain in manageable pieces. At this stage, you may become deeply saddened, angry, or consumed with guilt. Acknowledging these emotions is the key to recovery and acceptance of your loss. This process takes time: allowing yourself time to deal with your emotional wellbeing makes a lot of sense.

You and your partner You may feel and manage your loss very differently from your partner. By carrying your baby, you may have been much more aware of this new life than he was, and your loss may seem much more profound. In addition, you may mourn more openly and find strength in the support of others, whereas your partner may show much less emotion. Often men bury themselves in other tasks to manage their emotional pain. That does not mean that they don't care. Accepting these differences and communicating openly can help you both to grieve together and to begin planning a future pregnancy.

Rituals that bring closure Acknowledging that your baby was part of your life can be very helpful to the healing process. Rituals can be symbolic, such as a candlelight ceremony for you and your partner, or can include a physical memorial such as a special box. A memorial box can include an ultrasound photo, a baby outfit or other items, and writings – either a poem or your personal thoughts and feelings. Some women find that naming their lost child can make the loss more concrete and helps them to move on.

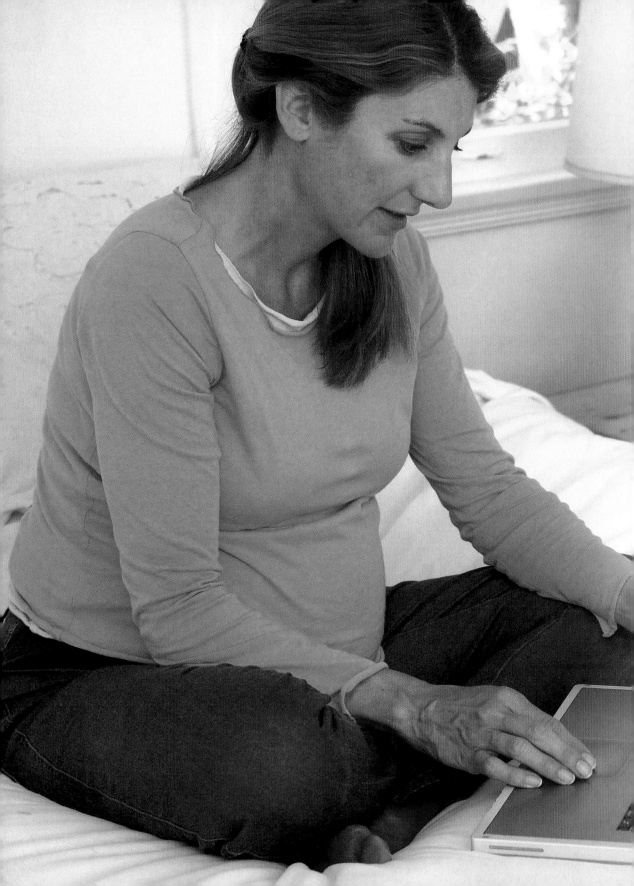

YOUR PREGNANCY

A PREGNANCY LATER IN LIFE IS LIKELY TO BE VERY **SPECIAL** AND **PRECIOUS** TO YOU. WHILE YOU MAY FEEL JUST AS EXCITED AS A WOMAN IN HER 20S, **YOUR EXPERIENCE** OF PREGNANCY MAY BE SOMEWHAT DIFFERENT. KNOWING HOW **YOUR BODY** WILL **REACT TO YOUR PREGNANCY**, AND **UNDERSTANDING WHAT TO DO** TO MAKE THE PREGNANCY AS **HEALTHY** AND **STRESS-FREE** AS POSSIBLE, WILL GO A LONG WAY TOWARDS MAKING YOUR EXPERIENCE **WHAT YOU WANT IT TO BE.**

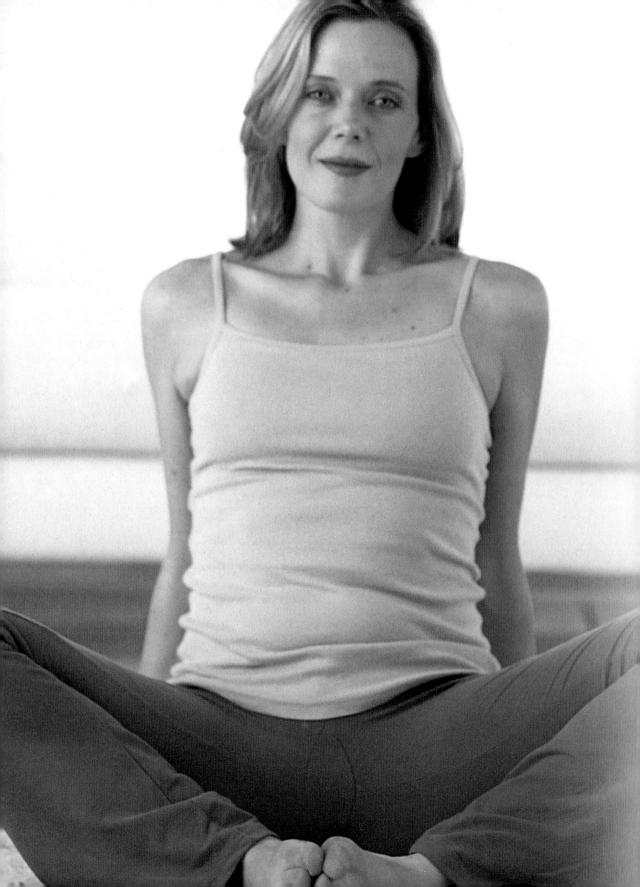

1ST TRIMESTER
what to expect

This is a time of huge change, both physical and emotional. While your body starts to create the environment for your baby to grow, you may feel exhausted and emotionally overwhelmed.

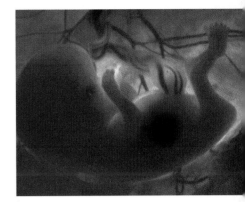

*This **9-week-old fetus** is already recognizably human. The limbs have formed and tiny fingers and toes are visible. Blood vessels are visible in the umbilical cord.*

PHYSICAL CHANGES

The most significant physical change in the early weeks of pregnancy is persistent tiredness, and although this feeling is by no means unique to women over 35, women who have had pregnancies in their 20s and again in their late 30s agree that the depth of fatigue is greater when older.

Many women also experience daily nausea or hunger pangs. The huge hormonal adjustments in response to pregnancy can also cause emotional turmoil. Being more tired than everyone else, and more irritable, introduces new challenges into your relationships and your career life.

During these first months of pregnancy, a gentle exercise programme can help restore your emotional balance and increase your energy. Your food plan will need to include meals that cover your increased requirements for protein and to help you deal with nausea (see pp48–49).

Now is also the time to meet the doctor or midwife who will care for you during the next 9 months and help bring your baby into the world. Understanding what to expect from your antenatal care will help you know what questions to ask your care provider and get the answers you need.

More screening and diagnostic tests are offered to women over 35 than to their younger counterparts. Becoming informed about tests, the pros and cons of genetic counselling, screening for Down syndrome (see pp56–57), and one of the earliest screening tests for developmental abnormalities, CVS (see pp58–59), will help ensure your experience is a positive one.

YOUR BABY

Your baby creates a life-sustaining connection with you, through the placenta. All of the major organs form during this time including your baby's heart, spine, and kidneys. Your baby's heart will start to beat, and the heartbeat can be seen on ultrasound by 6 weeks after your last period. Your baby's arms and legs will form and your baby will start to move although it is too early for you to feel it.

More tests are offered to **women over 35** than to their **younger counterparts**.

your body

Profound changes occur in your body within days of conceiving. In the first week you may feel surprisingly tired, and as the weeks go by you will notice increasing breast tenderness and probably one of the worst effects of early pregnancy – nausea. The changes in your body happen as a result of hormone levels that soar dramatically during pregnancy.

HORMONE CHANGES

Soon after conception, when the fertilized egg embeds in the lining of the uterus, the levels of two pregnancy hormones begin to rise. These hormones are progesterone, which is important in helping to maintain your pregnancy, and human chorionic gonadotropin (hCG). Progesterone has many effects on your body, one of which is to relax smooth muscle. We have this type of muscle in our internal organs such as the intestines and uterus. Smooth muscle relaxation is critical in pregnancy because the uterus must stretch, otherwise uterine contractions might cause preterm labour or miscarriage. You have a lot of other smooth muscles in your body that are also affected by progesterone. One of the first symptoms of progesterone you may notice is relaxation of your intestinal smooth muscle, which results in a lot of bloating and gas. Progesterone also profoundly affects the way you breathe, increasing how quickly you breathe and how deeply. Expect to feel short of breath when you walk up stairs, even if you are in good shape. Pregnancy hormones also make your breasts very sore, and they will start to enlarge.

The first trimester is also the beginning of a profound set of changes in your heart and circulation. The amount of blood pumping around your body starts to increase dramatically, and your heart has to work harder. As the uterus starts to enlarge it may press on the bladder, and you may feel the urge to pass urine more frequently than usual.

The exhaustion of early pregnancy is best dealt with by taking frequent naps if at all possible.

Dealing with Nausea

There are various approaches to help relieve nausea in pregnancy; try out a number of methods to find what works best for you.

- **Dietary changes** Some evidence suggests that small, protein-rich meals may help reduce nausea. Experiment with different foods to find the ones you tolerate best. You may need to avoid spicy foods, for example. It's important to snack in between feelings of nausea to avoid first trimester weight loss. Also, make sure you drink plenty of fluids. Don't worry too much about nutrition during the first few weeks; as long as you aren't losing weight, you are getting enough nutrition for the pregnancy. If you are losing weight, eat whatever you can keep down, and talk to your GP if your weight loss continues.

- **Medications** Several medications are helpful in alleviating nausea in pregnancy. The most important thing is to treat nausea early, instead of trying to tough it out. Delaying treatment may cause vomiting to become more severe over time. Taking pyridoxine (vitamin B$_6$) may help. Travel sickness tablets that contain promethazine have been used safely and successfully. Alternatively, taking ginger capsules (250mg) four times a day may help to reduce your symptoms. If none of these measures helps, ask your GP to prescribe an anti-sickness medication that is safe to use.

- **Acupressure** Acupressure bands have been marketed under many different names, but they are basically devices that are worn on the wrist to stimulate the P6 acupressure point. Inexpensive brands can be bought over the counter.

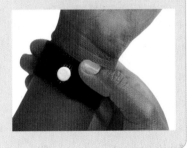

Even though this is annoying, don't be tempted to start drinking less fluids. Instead, go to the toilet regularly and wear clothes that are not a nightmare to get into and out of.

FEELING EXHAUSTED

Most women feel exhausted much of the time in these first few months. Although this is absolutely normal, it can be frustrating. Even if you are getting enough sleep, you may feel like you need a nap by 10am! This can make functioning at your job, or taking care of your family, feel particularly onerous.

In a perfect world you should give in to these feelings and take frequent naps. For many of us, this is not possible. If you can, allow yourself to slow down to whatever extent is possible. Don't feel guilty about going to sleep as early as you want to, and skip evening social events if you don't feel up to it. Let your partner organize meals, and pamper yourself whenever you can.

NAUSEA

Every pregnancy is different, but some nausea in pregnancy is common. About 50 per cent of women will have both nausea and vomiting, 25 per cent will have nausea only, and 25 per cent are unaffected. About two-thirds of women with severe nausea in a previous pregnancy will have similar symptoms in subsequent pregnancies. Taking an antenatal vitamin before conception may reduce the chance of nausea.

If nausea is so severe that you cannot hold down liquids, call your GP. Women with twins or triplets have higher levels of hormones and are more likely to experience nausea.

For most women, nausea starts to get better after the 12th week of pregnancy; however, early in pregnancy that light at the end of the tunnel can seem very far away. Only a small percentage of women continue to feel nauseous for their entire pregnancy. The one positive thing about nausea is that it is a sign of a healthy pregnancy.

your emotions

As your body undergoes tremendous physical changes to accommodate the growth of your baby, your pregnancy may uncover surprising emotions that challenge your self-image and comfort level. These physical and emotional changes can make you irritable and unhappy, and you may find it hard to relax during this trimester.

Early pregnancy is marked by changes in types and levels of hormones circulating in your body. For some women, fluctuating hormone levels have no discernable effects, but for others it can cause unpredictable emotional ups and downs that often defy explanation. If you are experiencing strong emotional upheavals, be assured that you are not "losing it" but are experiencing a sometimes disconcerting but normal adaptation to pregnancy.

DEALING WITH PHYSICAL CHANGES

Two common physical challenges of early pregnancy – exhaustion and nausea – are often difficult to handle. They have a direct impact on your everyday life and can accentuate your emotional highs and lows. Fatigue and continuous nausea can keep you from performing as well as usual at work, from getting things done at home, and from enjoying time with your partner and friends. Many women find it's best to resist the urge to fight these feelings. Allow yourself to slow down and rest as much as possible. Recognize that your body is undergoing incredible changes – you are accommodating the growth of another human being. Soothe yourself by remembering that your emotional volatility, low energy, and nausea are likely to start to recede after 12 weeks into your pregnancy. Accepting that this is a temporary stage may make you feel less guilty about getting the rest that you need. In a few months, you should be back to your usual schedule.

UNPLANNED PREGNANCIES

For women over 35, one in three pregnancies is unplanned, and in women over 40, this rises to as many as half. A surprise pregnancy may be very welcome news, but if it is not, it can be especially difficult when you are over 35. A late pregnancy imposes health risks you perhaps did not intend to take, and necessitates significant and possibly unwelcome changes in your career and personal life that may make you feel angry, hopeless, and depressed. Since you are reading this book, it's likely that you have decided to have your baby. Give yourself permission to grieve for the things you have to give up, but remember that you still have many choices. Motherhood is not the end of personal fulfilment for many women, and it doesn't have to be for you, either.

On Your Own

The first trimester, with its unpredictable emotions and physical changes, can be especially tough if you are not in a relationship. Pregnancy may seem to hit you head-on, and without support from a "significant other" you may begin to wonder whether you will be able to take care of yourself and your baby during the coming months. Remember that the first months are usually the most difficult ones. For now, try to reorganize your work schedule if you can (assuming you don't mind people knowing you are pregnant) to accommodate your need to rest. Try to find at least one support person who can help you when you are running really low on energy, and make a point of relaxing regularly.

RELAXATION

You can use relaxation to reduce stress in pregnancy, preserve your emotional resources, and manage pain during birth. Schedule some relaxation into your day, such as a lunch-time break in the park, or a ten-minute nap as soon as you get home from work. Short periods of regular relaxation throughout the day will help keep your energy levels up, and may help alleviate nausea in this physically challenging trimester.

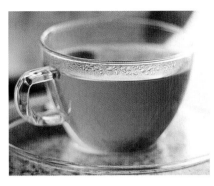

Herbal teas *offer good alternatives to caffeine and can be very relaxing.*

Breathing techniques Deep breathing is calming and soothing. The following breathing exercise can be done any time you feel stressed or tired. Set aside about 3 minutes and sit comfortably with your hands cradling your abdomen. Inhale through your nose for a count of four and feel your abdomen expand as your lungs fill with air and your diaphragm pushes down on your abdomen. Stop for an instant, then exhale through your mouth for a count of four. Slowly make your exhalations last two counts longer than your inhalations, to empty out the lungs fully before the next in-breath.

Imaging serenity Most people have a favourite place, perhaps somewhere in the mountains, at the beach, or near a childhood home. Imaging involves mentally visiting your special spot and resting there. This stimulates the secretion of serotonin in your brain, which makes you feel relaxed and positive. Schedule 5–15 minutes for your imaging session. Make sure to allow for a minute or two after your session to "come back" before rushing into your next activity.

Sit or lie down comfortably, close your eyes, and take a deep breath. Now imagine your favourite place, and that you are really there. If you are in the mountains, smell the flowers, hear the birds singing, and feel the soft, cool moss under your bare feet. When the time is up, open your eyes slowly and take a moment to enjoy feeling thoroughly relaxed. Sometimes imagery becomes easier when prompted with appropriate sounds or fragrances. Burning scented candles or listening to CDs with nature sounds, for example, can help take you to your favourite place.

Get a good night's sleep
When your energy level is low it is vital that you get plenty of sleep. You'll probably need more than you did before you were pregnant. Make time for extra sleep. It will make a valuable contribution to your emotional wellbeing.

Deep-breathing exercises can help you relax throughout pregnancy.

your relationships

During the first trimester of pregnancy, lack of energy, mood swings, and morning sickness are common and can change the dynamic of your relationships. You will want extra care from your partner, but because he cannot know exactly how you feel, you must communicate your needs to him. If you have other children, make sure you explain to them what is happening.

YOUR PARTNERSHIP

With significant physical and emotional changes taking place, you are likely to be very aware of your pregnancy in the first 3 months. However, not much has changed for your partner and he may find it difficult to understand how you are feeling.

Your partner's attitude Because he doesn't experience any physical changes himself, and since it is unlikely that you even look pregnant at this stage, your partner may have trouble comprehending the changes in your life and he might respond to you as

down on the amount of time you can spend together. Hormonal changes may make you feel suddenly overwhelmed emotionally, and you may begin to cry or snap at your partner without warning, which could confuse or upset him. In many ways you may not be as predictable and as much fun to be with as you used to be and that can be stressful for your partner.

Understanding each other Managing this huge life change together as a team will bring you closer. Because your emotions and physical wellness are difficult for your partner to predict or discern, it helps

to help your partner **understand your needs,** explain how you experience the changes in your body

he would normally. Many men seem forgetful of, and impatient with, their pregnant partner's need to rest and be given special consideration. If this describes your partner, you may feel misunderstood and unappreciated.

In order to be supportive, your partner may need to make some adjustments. Depending on how much your pregnancy has affected you, he may need to learn to live with a brand new you. For instance, to control nausea, you may have to get up slowly in the morning while he races along as usual. You may be too tired to participate in the sports you played together, or have to go to bed earlier at night, cutting

if you openly share your feelings and communicate your needs. Explain to him that you need more compassion and nurturing from him than usual. After all, you are carrying the bulk of the burden of parenthood right now. Many men can't guess what makes their partners feel better, while independent, self-sufficient women may find it hard to admit that they have exhausted their own resources. However, informing your partner early on of your need to rest, and being prepared to ask for help with specific household tasks that might normally fall to you, will give him the opportunity to support you during these challenging months.

Low energy Your lower energy level is a predictable fact of early pregnancy. Therefore, your routine will have to be adjusted. Instead of arguing over who will handle household tasks as they come up, sit down with your partner and consider the priorities you have as a couple. This will clarify which activities are important to you and which ones can be cut out right away. Sometimes a compromise is more easily reached if you agree to eliminate an activity for a certain time or to alternate between activities and tasks.

Surprise babies Remaining united as a couple is particularly important if neither of you has planned for this pregnancy. Difficult times are usually easier managed together, and this teamwork can strengthen your relationship. Most couples also find that, after the first shock, they are able to share the challenge of adjusting to a new baby in their lives and begin to look forward to becoming parents.

Sex during the first trimester Many couples wonder whether having sex during pregnancy can lead to miscarriage. Men often are afraid that they will hurt their baby during intercourse. However, in a normal healthy pregnancy, neither of these fears is necessary. Remember that your doctor or midwife is a reliable resource for any questions concerning sex during your pregnancy. Don't be embarrassed to ask them these questions – they are very commonly asked during pregnancy.

Some women do experience a decrease in libido during the first trimester. Obviously, exhaustion, painful breasts, and nausea do not incite a burning desire for sex. Cuddling can become an important temporary substitute for the intimacy that you used to share by making love. A little gentle attention may even put you in the mood for sex.

YOUR OTHER CHILDREN

If you already have children and are juggling the double duty of career and motherhood, the first trimester can be overwhelming. Your children will notice your fatigue, nausea, and impatience quickly. Younger children often become frightened at the thought that their mother is not well, especially if there is no apparent reason. It is a good idea to acknowledge that you are very tired while reassuring your child that soon you will definitely be fine again.

Remember that your partner can be a great source of comfort to your child if you are unable to spend as much time with him or her as usual, or can't play as energetically as you did previously.

Teenagers can be a special challenge when you are dealing with fluctuating hormones yourself. It may be best to inform your teenage child of your pregnancy early on. He or she may react by acting disgusted or unaffected, but once adjusted to the idea, he or she may feel excited about becoming involved.

Time with dad can help make up for the fact that mum isn't feeling well enough to play today.

your career

For many women, the first trimester is the most difficult time at work – battling fatigue and nausea much of the time while perhaps trying to hide this from employers and colleagues. There are several practical measures you can take to help you get through these months.

STAYING SAFE AND COMFORTABLE AT WORK

The excitement of being pregnant can dissipate with the onslaught of morning sickness and fatigue that accompanies early pregnancy for many women. This is particularly true if you are trying to maintain your composure at work, especially if no one knows you are pregnant. There are measures you can take to keep as comfortable – and therefore as productive – as possible, and also to take care of your growing baby.

Morning sickness For some women, nausea can last all day. Your diet (see p48–49) and some medical interventions (see p38–39) can help control morning

If you can fulfil as many of your usual tasks and responsibilities, and maintain as much productivity as possible, your pregnancy is more likely to be well-received. Maintaining your professionalism during this important life-experience will help get the message across to your boss and colleagues that your career is also important to you. A favourable impression early on will set the stage for their attitude towards you after pregnancy, boosting their confidence in your continued productivity and success in the long term.

Towards the end of your pregnancy, when you will need to slow down, your co-workers and boss are

despite the **allowances** you have to make, being pregnant doesn't stop you from being **a reliable professional**

sickness. If you have trouble getting started in the morning, you may be able to negotiate coming to work an hour later and staying later in the evening, to avoid the rush-hour congestion. Grazing throughout the day on tasty high-protein snacks, such as nuts, trail mix, some cheese, or even a milkshake may help your symptoms. Keep alert for smells that cause you to become nauseated so you can avoid them as much as possible.

Lack of energy Many women find the lack of energy in early pregnancy overwhelming. Make sure you do all you can to maintain energy.

likely to be more understanding if they feel you have done your best to continue to be a valuable asset throughout your pregnancy.

Take a balanced view about maintaining your productivity at work, and listen to your body. If you are exhausted, then slow down. Remember you will probably feel much better and more energized in the next trimester and can catch up with things then. Rest as much as possible to support the extra workload your body is doing in supporting the development and growth of your baby.

Having small, healthy snacks throughout the day will maintain your energy. In addition, take small breaks and relax your body and mind with two or three deep breaths. Take your entire lunch break and enjoy a good rest in the middle of the day.

Try to leave work on time at night, so that you have as much time as possible to relax and enjoy your partner's company. Go to bed early enough to get plenty of sleep each night – this will also help you to maintain your energy levels.

Work stress may be unavoidable, but is exhausting, and will deplete your energy. Do all that you can to minimize your everyday stresses. Regular exercise and a good diet can help, as can pampering yourself with massage and reflexology.

DEALING WITH YOUR BOSS

If you have told people at work that you are pregnant, you may become aware of how accommodating your boss, your colleagues, or your company's parenting policies are, or how inflexibly and impersonally the needs of new parents are handled. This may provide a completely new perspective of your workplace and gives you a glimpse of the professional environment into which you may have to integrate your parenting goals. How your company meets your needs early in pregnancy is usually indicative of how your requests will be met as a parent in the future.

Timing the announcement You are obliged to notify your employer of your pregnancy and intention to take maternity leave by the end of the 15th week before your expected week of childbirth. Many women wait until the end of the first trimester to tell their boss. By then the risk of miscarriage is low, and you may have already had first trimester screening for chromosomal abnormalities (see p54) and/or CVS (see p58) showing a normal pregnancy. If you suffer from overwhelming fatigue or morning sickness, or if your job is very stressful, speak with your boss earlier so you can negotiate adjustments to your schedule that will help you to be more comfortable and productive. Your timing may depend on how your boss has handled previous pregnancies in your company. If you expect an unfavourable

reaction, wait until you have demonstrated your productivity as a pregnant employee. Immediately after the successful completion of a project, for example, would make a perfect occasion to connect your pregnancy with your ability to work well.

Considering the needs of your boss and colleagues Make sure you are informed about your maternity leave options (see p14–15) and approach your boss with a plan for your transition out of work, time away, and return to work. Most bosses will appreciate that you have thought not only of your own needs but also of those of your colleagues and company. This may put you in a favourable position to negotiate flexible work hours during your pregnancy.

Since your job will be held during your absence, your colleagues may be the recipients of your assignments when you leave. They may wonder whether you will return to work and take back your workload. Assure them that you are aware of their concerns and interested in smooth transitions for all involved.

Tips for Working Mums-to-be

Certain practical measures can make a significant difference to the way you feel at work, and consequently, your productivity. Try the following tips.

- Break your lunch hour into more frequent, shorter breaks of 15 to 20 minutes.
- Rest during your breaks. Close your eyes and allow yourself to cat nap.
- Keep a supply of snacks at work. Frequent snacking helps combat nausea in the first trimester.
- Keep a glass of water handy and drink throughout the day. Try to empty your glass at least four times during an 8-hour day and go to the toilet frequently.
- Try walking around as much as possible to increase circulation, reduce swelling, and prevent blood clots in your legs, which are more common in pregnancy.
- If you stand up for most of the day, try and get some time sitting down, with your feet up, during every hour.

exercise programme

During the first months of pregnancy, it is important to heed your body's signals and slow down. Even though there are few visible changes, your body is handling immense adjustments. Adding too much exercise can dangerously deplete your physical and emotional resources, so exercise in moderation.

During pregnancy, being active for 30 minutes each day will provide many benefits – stress reduction, improved sleep, hormonal (and, therefore, emotional) balance, increased energy, physical fitness, and reduced pregnancy symptoms. Women who exercise regularly have better posture, which helps them alleviate or avoid back pain. They also tend to suffer less from swelling and bloating and gain less weight during pregnancy than women who don't exercise.

If you are starting to exercise, consider gentle activities such as walking, yoga, or pregnancy exercise classes. Having fun and seeing progress are both great motivators for continuing with an exercise programme, and regular exercise is the key to a beneficial regimen. Before you begin, ask your doctor to approve your programme.

INTENSITY AND DURATION

Make sure your workouts energize you. If, at the end of your workout, you feel tired and discouraged, exercise less vigorously and less frequently. Alter any existing regime to suit your pregnant state.

Finding the right intensity

You should be able to talk without feeling breathless when doing gentle exercise (especially if you were unfit before pregnancy). This will be difficult during aerobic activity. If you have a heart-rate monitor, keep to your target heart rate (see opposite).

Gentle activities, such as yoga stretches, are ideal exercises for pregnancy.

Duration Limit aerobic workouts to 30 minutes, with adequate warm-up and cool-down periods. Non-aerobic exercise (such as weight training) can be done for up to an hour, as long as it is gentle. During non-aerobic exercises, drink juices to maintain your blood sugar levels if necessary.

TARGET HEART RATE

To exercise safely and effectively, you need to calculate your maximum heart rate (MHR), and from this, your target heart rate for pregnancy. MHR is calculated by subtracting your age from 220. In pregnancy, a goal of 60–80 per cent of MHR is acceptable. In women who are out of shape, a target heart rate of 50–60 per cent of MHR is a good limit. In fit women, a target heart rate of 70–80 per cent of MHR is safe. For example, if you are age 35 and were fit before pregnancy, you should exercise most energetically at between 130–148 beats per minute. If you were out of shape before pregnancy, this should be reduced to 93–111 beats a minute.

EXERCISING SAFELY

Avoid overheating, which may be detrimental to your baby's central nervous system development in this trimester. Wear loose clothing and a well-fitting sports bra. Drink water at least 30 minutes before your workout and during your workout. Do not perform energetic exercise if you have a fever, or in hot, humid conditions. Do not exercise to exhaustion. Heed your body's warning signals and, at any stage of pregnancy, stop exercising at once and call your hospital if you experience:

- uncomfortable or frequent contractions not near the due date
- vaginal bleeding or leaking of amniotic fluid
- headaches that do not go away
- skipped or very rapid heart beats
- dizziness
- decrease or cessation of your baby's movements
- increased shortness of breath
- extreme muscle weakness
- calf pain or swelling.

Exercises to avoid during pregnancy include contact sports, scuba diving, gymnastics, horse riding, and downhill or water skiing. Avoid any exercise that involves a risk of impact or falling.

IDEAL EXERCISES FOR THE 1ST TRIMESTER

Exercise	Benefits and suggestions	Frequency and duration
Walking	Walking can be adjusted to your daily energy level. You can choose your environment – a peaceful park or a busy street – to match your needs. And you can ask a friend or your partner to come along.	A daily 20–30 minute walk is great, if you can.
Cycling	If you like cycling, make the most of it in your first trimester – cycling gets tricky later because your belly gets in the way and balance becomes less reliable. Use a path and remember to wear a helmet.	Two to three times a week for 20–30 minutes.
Low-impact step classes	The company of others and a firm time commitment are motivators. You will be in climate-controlled, comfortable conditions throughout the year. Adjusting the height of your step sets your workout intensity.	Two to three times a week for no more than 45 minutes.
Yoga	Slow, gentle yoga moves can help you breathe deeply and relax. As you carefully control your exercise through the entire range of motion, you will strengthen your muscles and improve your flexibility.	Daily for gentle workouts; or 3 times a week.

food plan

During this trimester, you begin to "eat for two". This doesn't mean eating as much as two people – you'll need little more than you ate prior to pregnancy. However, make sure your diet is rich in protein, vitamins, and minerals to provide your baby with the essential building blocks needed for development.

VITAL NUTRIENTS

What you eat will, to some extent, determine how well your baby develops during pregnancy. A well-balanced diet will provide your baby with all the nutrients needed for healthy development.

Protein Throughout pregnancy, women should have at least 60g of protein in their daily diet, and women over 35 need an additional 4–5g. Protein provides the building blocks for your growing uterus, placenta, and breasts and your baby's developing tissues. Include some high protein foods into your diet daily (see opposite).

Iron Your iron requirement during pregnancy doubles to 30mg. Iron is needed for the formation of red blood cells, and you will need sufficient iron stores from the start of your pregnancy to maintain a good energy level. Anaemia (low iron levels) can leave you exhausted during pregnancy and too weak to handle the demands of labour.

Chicken salad is a delicious light meal. It provides you with plenty of nutrients and is full of protein.

Eating foods that are rich in iron (see opposite) will help you maintain energy throughout this physically challenging trimester.

Many women begin pregnancy with an inadequate iron level. The increased need for iron during pregnancy can make it difficult to get the iron needed from food alone. In such cases, doctors recommend taking extra iron on top your prenatal supplements.

Vitamin and mineral supplements

Even though your vitamin requirements rise in pregnancy, excessive supplement doses can be dangerous. Megadoses of the fat-soluble vitamins A and D, for example, are thought to be harmful to your baby. Specially formulated preparations for pregnancy contain reduced doses of these vitamins. Do not take supplements that are not designed for pregnancy. Ask your healthcare provider for a recommendation.

FOODS TO AVOID

There are certain foods pregnant women should avoid because of the risks of food-borne diseases, such as toxoplasmosis, E. coli, and listeriosis, that can harm your baby.

Toxoplasmosis is caused by a parasite. It is not dangerous to you, but can harm your baby if you

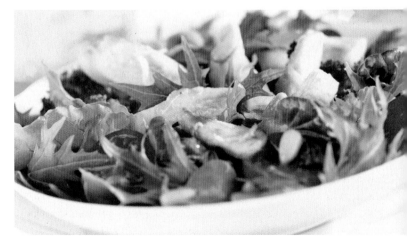

come into contact with it during pregnancy or just before you conceive, causing birth defects.

Listeriosis is caused by a bacteria, which can cross the placenta and infect your baby. Infection can cause miscarriage, or premature delivery, and even fetal death. Pregnant women are more likely than other adults to develop listeriosis, so you should avoid foods that could potentially be contaminated (see below).

Salmonella poisoning is unlikely to cause any damage to your baby. However, it will seriously deplete your resources during a time when your body is already taxed.

Undercooked meat or uncooked meat or fish Eating these foods puts you at risk of exposure to food-borne bacteria such as E. coli and salmonella. Avoid uncooked seafood as well as rare or uncooked meat or poultry.

Ready-to-eat meats Deli meats can be contaminated with listeria. Eat only if you can heat them thoroughly. Avoid hot dogs and pâté, which can contain listeria.

Liver and other organ meats Vitamin A is found in substantial quantities in liver and large amounts of this vitamin have been linked with birth defects. Offal, such as liver and kidney, often contain the highest levels of toxins in an animal's body. For this reason it's best not to eat any offal while you are pregnant.

Unpasteurized milk Drink only milk that has been pasteurized. Unpasteurized milk could be contaminated with listeria.

Soft cheeses These might contain listeria. Stick to cheese made with pasteurized milk. Avoid imported soft cheeses such as camembert, brie, and gorgonzola.

Raw eggs Eating undercooked or raw eggs risks exposure to salmonella. Avoid foods that may contain raw egg, such as Caesar dressing, mayonnaise, and Hollandaise sauce.

Fish exposed to pollutants Dangerous levels of mercury have been detected in certain fish, which can affect your baby's brain development. Fish to avoid are marlin, shark, and swordfish. You should also minimize the amount of tuna you eat. (See also p21.)

DIET AND MORNING SICKNESS Many women experience nausea in this trimester and this nausea is almost bound to affect your appetite. Some women are affected all day. Try the following tips to help overcome this nausea and get the nutrients you need.

- Eat low-fat, high-carbohydrate foods, such as crackers, cereal, or plain toast.
- Eat small amounts of protein-rich foods.
- Eat small meals supplemented by frequent, nutritious snacks.
- Drink plenty of water.

Sources of Protein

The following foods are rich sources of protein and are good to eat during pregnancy.

- Meat such as lean beef, lamb, pork, and chicken.
- Fish and seafood (but avoid fish that may be contaminated with mercury, see p 21).
- Dairy products, such as milk, yogurt, cheese, and eggs.
- Beans and pulses, such as lentils, kidney beans, lima beans, baked beans, and chickpeas.
- Seeds and nuts.
- Tofu and soy products.
- Cereals, such as muesli, and brown rice contain some protein.

Sources of Iron

Iron is important for red blood cell formation and you need twice as much as you did before you became pregnant. The following foods are good sources of iron.

- Red meat, especially beef.
- Poultry, dark meat.
- Eggs.
- Dried fruits such as apricots, prunes, and figs.
- Green leafy vegetables: broccoli, kale, turnip greens, and spinach.
- Fortified cereals.
- Seeds and nuts, such as cashew nuts and sunflower seeds.
- Pulses such as lentils, chickpeas, and kidney beans.

antenatal care

In the first trimester, your first task is to decide who you want to look after you during your pregnancy and deliver your baby. This is a big decision and is linked with the type of birth you want to have. There are several options for choosing who will look after you during your pregnancy.

CHOOSING WHO WILL PROVIDE ANTENATAL CARE

One of the most popular strategies for choosing a care provider is to talk to friends who have had babies in the last couple of years, although in many areas choice may be limited by distance. Another approach is to decide where you want to deliver: a hospital, a free-standing birth centre, or at home. Most women will be referred to their local hospital by their GP and will be cared for by a combination of GP, midwife, and consultant obstetrician. Low-risk women may not see a consultant at all, but have their care given in their home or GP surgery by GPs and midwives.

Consultant-led care Doctors may view birth as uncomplicated for most women, but are more likely than midwives to be sensitized to the development of potential medical problems; this focus on the medical aspects of pregnancy has pros and cons for women over the age of 35. If you prefer to be cared for by an obstetrician, you have the option but will probably see the midwives, too.

Midwife-led care Midwives view pregnancy and birth as an uncomplicated fact of everyday life. Usually they look after only low-risk patients, but most midwives will not consider you to be high risk just because you are over the age of 35. However, if you are having more than one baby, have a significant medical problem, or have had a prior Caesarean delivery you are not a good candidate for midwife care. Many midwives work in groups to give continuity of care. Midwife care usually pairs with hospital birth and one of the team may deliver you, if this service is available.

Independent midwives have elected to provide a private service to women and may work alone or in groups. The service is expensive but highly personalized with care timed to suit the pregnant woman. Scans will usually be arranged with a private obstetrician and the independent midwife will be on call to attend the labour and delivery. Delivery may be in a local hospital (often by special arrangement), in a birth centre, or at the woman's home. Independent midwives tend to favour natural childbirth and if

a woman seeking private care needs medical supervision of her pregnancy she may choose to see a private obstetrician and deliver in a private maternity unit.

Shared care This refers to a pattern of care shared between the hospital and the GP, which has been largely superseded by midwife/GP-led care.

CHOOSING WHERE TO DELIVER

In general, your choice of where you deliver will determine your care provider. The majority of doctors take care of women in hospital settings, where most UK births take place. Midwives mainly take care of women in a hospital setting, although they also deliver babies in birth centres or at home.

Hospital birth There are three potential advantages to choosing to deliver in hospital. First, if you are among the 30–40 per cent of women over 35 who require a Caesarean delivery, there will be no need for you to be moved from home or the birth centre. The second advantage is that you will have more pain control options.

Although many first-time mothers wish to avoid epidural analgesia, you may not know what type of pain relief you want until you are actually in labour. If you are determined to avoid epidural analgesia (see pp128–129), freestanding birth centres and home birth are geared towards supporting you without pain medicine. A third advantage is that a hospital birth may be safer if you have significant medical problems such as diabetes or blood pressure problems, which may affect you or your baby. It is also safest to deliver in a hospital if you've had a Caesarean section previously because of the small risk of the uterus rupturing.

Birth centre or home birth If you are having a normal, healthy pregnancy, the risks when giving birth in an alternative setting are low. Delivery at a birth centre may increase your chances of avoiding intervention during labour. In addition, because epidural analgesia is not usually available, you are likely to receive more intensive labour support for your pain.

NHS community midwives will usually be able to advise women who wish to give birth at home. This service is available in most areas and groups of midwives will usually cover each other on a rota basis. Home birth is an option for those who prefer to avoid the use of painkilling drugs and who wish to keep intervention to a minimum. The midwife will

discuss in advance the management of emergencies and possible transfer into hospital.

GETTING THE MOST FROM YOUR ANTENATAL CARE

It is important that you feel comfortable with your choice of antenatal care. Your midwife will be able to answer your questions or will refer you to an obstetrician for further discussion. All hospitals will be able to tell you their Caesarean delivery or episiotomy rate, but this may be influenced by their patient population and by the level of care they provide for newborn babies (a hospital that looks after babies from 24 weeks will probably have a higher Caesarean rate than one which only looks after babies from 32 weeks).

Finding a doctor or midwife who makes you comfortable and who shares a similar philosophy about pregnancy and birth is important.

your first appointment

Your first visit with a care provider is important. During this visit, he or she will take a full medical history to determine if you have any underlying health problems. In addition, your provider will ask you about any health problems that run in your family, and in your partner's family.

Unless you have a preexisting medical problem, your doctor will usually treat you like any other pregnant woman in terms of scheduling your first appointment, at about 8 weeks. One of the main reasons for the delay is that early miscarriage is very common and in most cases cannot be prevented by medical treatment. Therefore, most providers wait until you have passed the danger zone of early miscarriage before they order all the pregnancy blood tests.

PREPARING FOR YOUR APPOINTMENT

If your partner is not going to come with you to your first visit, it's important for you to sit down together and brainstorm about possible family problems. Any family conditions may be passed on to your baby, and testing may be an option.

If you have any health problems, such as high blood pressure or diabetes, bring your medical records with you. Your questions can then be answered right away instead of having to wait until your provider can get copies of your records. You may

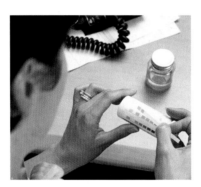

A urine sample will help provide information about any undiagnosed infection or diabetes.

get asked some embarrassing but important questions about drug use, sexually transmitted diseases, and past pregnancy terminations. It's critical that you tell the truth about your medical history. If your partner doesn't know about it, you can arrange to tell your provider when your partner is not present.

STANDARD TESTS

In addition to answering a lot of questions, your doctor will probably give you a thorough physical examination as well as measuring your height and weight. Your doctor should also discuss your options for first trimester screening for

abnormalities so that tests can be arranged between 10–14 weeks if you want them (see pp54–59). Depending on how many weeks pregnant you are, you may get to hear your baby's heartbeat. Finally, you will be asked to give samples of your blood and urine for routine testing and you will also have your blood pressure checked (see opposite).

ADDITIONAL TESTS

As well as these routine tests you may also have some additional tests, depending on your personal medical history. It is likely your doctor will arrange for you to have an ultrasound scan to determine the exact number of weeks you are pregnant and to exclude twins or a "silent" miscarriage (where the baby has died but there have been no symptoms). This scan is usually done between 8 and 12 weeks.

You may also have a blood test to check for HIV (the virus that causes AIDS). Testing for HIV is now recommended for all pregnant women. If you have HIV, the chances of passing the virus on to your baby can be greatly reduced by taking antiretroviral agents.

ROUTINE TESTS

Blood tests

- **Full blood count** This test screens for anaemia, which is very common during pregnancy. Anaemia may be due to low iron levels, or can be an inherited form, such as thalassaemia.
- **Blood type** This test will determine your blood type (A, B, O, or AB) as well as show if you are Rhesus positive (Rh+) or negative (Rh-). If you are Rhesus negative, you will usually receive a medication called anti-D after any medical procedure, such as amniocentesis, or if you have vaginal bleeding. You will usually get an extra dose at around 28 and 34 weeks.
- **Antibody screen** This test determines whether you have antibodies that could cross the placenta and cause the baby to become anaemic.
- **Hepatitis B** This test will identify women who are actively infectious with hepatitis B, a viral liver disease that can be transmitted to the baby during pregnancy and labour.
- **Rubella** This blood test determines whether you are immune to rubella. If you are not, you will usually get vaccinated right after delivery. You cannot have the vaccine during pregnancy.
- **Syphilis** This sexually transmitted disease does not always cause symptoms in the mother but it can cause serious problems for the fetus.

Urine test

This test looks for protein in your urine, and for signs of a urinary tract infection (UTI). Extra protein in the urine can be a sign of kidney disease. UTIs will be treated with antibiotics to prevent a serious kidney infection, which can cause pregnancy complications.

Blood pressure

Blood pressure usually falls in the middle of pregnancy. Women with high or high normal blood pressure early in pregnancy are at increased risk of having blood pressure problems later.

Weight

This baseline value will let your care provider calculate how much weight you have gained as your pregnancy progresses. Many hospitals only weigh women at their first visit.

If you are uncertain as to whether you have had chickenpox, you should stay away from people with this infectious disease while you are pregnant. If you have no immunity and do happen to be exposed, there is treatment to prevent severe chickenpox from developing during pregnancy.

If you are of Afro–Caribbean, African, Mediterranean, or Hispanic descent you will have tests for the blood disorders sickle cell anaemia or thalassaemia.

YOUR DUE DATE

Last but not least you will be given your due date at your booking appointment. This date is sometimes referred to as the EDD or estimated date of delivery.

Your due date is based on your last menstrual period. Even if you think you know when you conceived, your last menstrual period is the most accurate way of estimating your due date. The exception occurs when you don't remember when your last period

was or you have very irregular periods. Then an early ultrasound will be the most accurate way to date your pregnancy. Don't get too attached to your due date – remember it is only an estimate. Usually your doctor or midwife will see you again in 4–6 weeks time to review your test results and discuss first trimester screening results. However, your doctor or midwife should call you before your second visit if any of the results are abnormal.

screening for abnormalities

As women age there is an increased risk of having a baby with problems caused by extra or missing chromosomes. Over recent years, tests to detect the risk of these conditions have improved and become more accurate and more widely available. However, the decision to be tested, and which test to have is still a matter of individual choice.

CHROMOSOME ABNORMALITIES

Screening tests in this trimester are directed towards looking for chromosome abnormalities in your baby. The most well-known abnormality is Down syndrome, caused by the presence of an extra chromosome 21. The risk of chromosome abnormalities occurring increases noticeably as we age, and is particularly marked once you get into your 40s. Screening for neural tube defects does not happen until the second trimester (see p76–77).

Down syndrome is caused by the presence of an extra chromosome 21. The degree of disability is variable, but all babies with Down syndrome have some degree of learning difficulties. Heart defects and poor vision are common.

Trisomy 18 is caused by an extra copy of chromosome 18 and affects about 1 in 3,000 live births. While many fetuses with trisomy 18 will die before birth, survivors can live for several years with profound mental retardation. Most fetuses with trisomy 18 will have significant abnormalities that can be seen on ultrasound.

Trisomy 13 affects about 1 in 5,000 live births, and is caused by the presence of an extra copy of chromosome 13. Most fetuses with trisomy 13 have abnormalities that can be detected on ultrasound, including heart defects, cleft lip, and brain abnormalities. Most babies with trisomy 13 die within 3 months after birth.

Turner syndrome occurs when a female fetus is missing all or part of one of her X chromosomes. Unlike the other trisomies, Turner syndrome is not more common as women age. Malformations are common and may include heart defects and kidney problems. Most affected pregnancies end in miscarriage; however, around 1 in 2,500 girls has this condition. They are usually short and unable to have their own children.

Klinefelter syndrome occurs when a male baby has an extra X sex chromosome. It occurs in 1 in 500 to 1 in 800 live male births. Boys with Klinefelter syndrome have developmental problems, especially receptive language delay, despite overall average to above average intelligence.

DECIDING TO BE TESTED

Whether to have screening tests for abnormalities is a personal choice. One of the first things many women consider is how they

RISK OF CHROMOSOMAL ABNORMALITIES						
Maternal age at EDD	30	35	38	42	44	46
Risk of Down syndrome at birth	1 in 952	1 in 385	1 in 175	1 in 64	1 in 38	1 in 23
Risk of any abnormality at birth	1 in 384	1 in 204	1 in 103	1 in 40	1 in 25	1 in 15

FIRST TRIMESTER TEST OPTIONS

Name of test	Result given	How the test works
1st trimester blood test (see p56)	Estimated risk of Down syndrome or trisomy 18	Blood sample tested for two hormone levels. When combined with the result of the nuchal transluceny test it gives an estimate of the risk of Down syndrome.
Nuchal translucency scan (see p57)	Estimated risk of Down syndrome	Ultrasound scan measures the thickness of a fold of skin at the back of the baby's neck. The scan is often combined with a blood test.
Chorionic villus sampling (CVS, see pp58–59)	Definitive diagnosis of Down syndrome or other chromosome abnormality	Sample of placental tissue is taken by one of two procedures and chromosomes analysed in the laboratory.

would use the information once they have it. A crucial point is that there is no cure for chromosomal abnormalities. If you find out that your baby is affected, you will have only two choices: to continue with the pregnancy or not to.

This is likely to be a very tough decision. Some women are sure they would continue with their pregnancy no matter what problems are found. Others feel strongly that they would have a termination. However, most women are unsure about what decision they would make. Until you are faced with the situation, have learnt all you can about the problem, and thought about what it would mean for your baby and your family, it's hard to know what you would do.

Even for women who plan to continue their pregnancy knowing the fetus is abnormal, testing may carry some benefits. Women who know their baby's diagnosis before

birth often have a more positive experience when they come to deliver their babies. They have had time to learn about their baby's condition, talk to other mothers, join support groups, and prepare their families. For this reason no one should rule out testing without considering all the pros and cons.

TEST OPTIONS

If you decide to be tested there are two options: non-invasive screening tests and definitive tests. For example, your age itself is a kind of screening test providing you with an initial risk of chromosome problems (see opposite). First trimester screening combines your age with the results of a blood test and an ultrasound test. Second trimester screening combines your age with a blood test. Both of these tests yield a personal risk profile, which may be higher or

lower than your original risk based on your age.

The major drawback to non-invasive tests is that they do not give you a definitive result. In other words, it cannot tell you if your child has Down syndrome, only a numerical risk of whether he or she may or not. The only way to find out for sure is to have a definitive invasive test – either chorionic villus sampling (CVS, see pp58–59) in the first trimester or amniocentesis (see pp78–79) at 15–18 weeks. Both of these tests carry a small risk of miscarriage.

Women over 35 are often given the option of moving directly to one of these tests. However, some women start with one of the screening tests to see if their risk of having a baby with defects drops significantly. If it does, you may no longer want to take the risk of having an invasive test that carries the chance of miscarriage.

first trimester screening

For women who want information about the risk of Down syndrome but wish to avoid moving directly to an invasive test such as chorionic villus sampling (CVS, see pp58–59) or amniocentesis (see pp80–81), first trimester testing offers an early screening option, but cannot give a definitive result.

First trimester screening is performed between 10 and 13 weeks of pregnancy and uses a combination of a blood test and an ultrasound to determine the risk of your baby being born with Down syndrome or some other chromosome abnormality. The ultrasound measures the thickness of the skin at the back of your baby's neck, called the nuchal fold, which is thicker in babies with Down syndrome. On the same day as the scan, you may have blood taken and tested for levels of pregnancy-associated plasma protein-A (PAPP-A) and human chorionic gonadotropin (hCG). Using the combined results of blood tests, age, and nuchal translucency measurement, the doctor will be able to calculate your baby's risk of Down syndrome. You will receive the results a few days after the test. Your risk will be compared with what the risk of chromosomal abnormality would be for a woman of your age. Your new risk

An ultrasound scan in the first trimester can help reassure you that all is well with your baby.

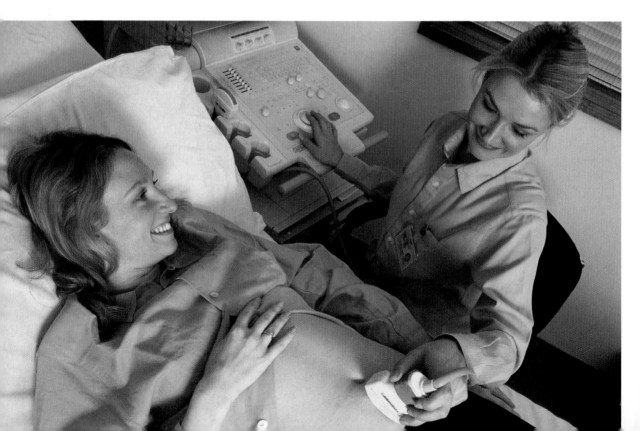

Nuchal Translucency Scan

The test is usually performed at 11–14 weeks of pregnancy. The doctor or technician (sonographer) performing the scan will place the ultrasound probe on your tummy and look for an area at the back of the baby's neck called the nuchal translucency.

The person doing the scan will mark two points and take a measurement of the thickness at this point.

If the measurement is small, the risk of Down syndrome is low (the exact measurement depends on the size of the baby). A larger thickness at this point generally indicates that there is a higher than normal risk of the baby having Down syndrome.

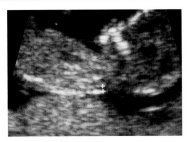

Normal nuchal scan *shows the outline of the baby, two crosses marking the back of the neck. A narrow gap suggests a low risk of Down syndrome.*

The nuchal translucency scan result must be combined with the results of your blood tests to assess accurately your baby's risk of Down syndrome.

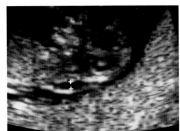

Abnormal scan *shows a thickening at the back of the neck (marked with two crosses). The greater the thickness, the higher the risk of Down syndrome.*

This test is very dependent on the skill of the sonographer. A poor ultrasound can miss Down syndrome or give a "positive" result with a normal baby.

may be higher, lower, or the same as your risk based on your age alone. The test is called "positive" if your risk of having a baby with Down syndrome is higher than a pre-set cutoff point, usually 1 in 250. A positive test does not mean that your baby has Down syndrome, only that your risk is greater. First trimester screening will also detect most babies affected by trisomy 18.

TEST ACCURACY

In women over the age of 35, first trimester screening will detect 85–95 per cent of babies with Down syndrome. However, it can also give a "false negative" result (suggesting the baby is at low risk of Down syndrome when in fact the baby is affected). First

trimester screening will be negative in between 5 and 15 per cent of pregnancies where the baby has Down syndrome.

HOW AGE AFFECTS RESULTS

The test is more likely to come back positive as you get older. In women over the age of 35, a

quarter of tests will be "positive". Although most of these mothers will still have a normal baby, their results may make CVS or amniocentesis a reasonable option. However, 75 per cent of women will have a negative test and can feel more comfortable about avoiding CVS or amniocentesis.

RESULTS

If your test is positive Even with a "positive" result, the chance of your baby having Down syndrome is still very small. You will be told the actual statistical risk of your baby having Down syndrome; you can compare this risk to the risk of miscarriage with CVS or amniocentesis. Only one of these tests can give you a definitive answer.

If your test is negative If your first trimester screening test is negative, then your baby has a very, very low chance of having Down syndrome. However, if you are still nervous after the screening test, you can have either CVS or amniocentesis. Both of these tests will give you a definitive result.

chorionic villus sampling

Many women now have the option of having earlier testing to determine whether their baby has Down syndrome. In chorionic villus sampling, a small fragment of the placenta is removed for chromosomal analysis. The advantage of this test is that it can be done up to 5 weeks earlier than amniocentesis.

The technique of chorionic villus sampling (CVS) has become an increasingly popular method of checking for chromosome abnormalities at a much earlier stage than amniocentesis. It is usually done between 10 and 14 weeks of pregnancy.

WHAT IS CVS?

During CVS, a small amount of tissue is carefully removed from your placenta for analysis. Because the placenta develops from the fertilized egg, chromosomes in cells from this tissue are the same as your baby's chromosomes.

CVS will tell you if your baby has a chromosomal disorder such as Down syndrome. It will not detect neural tube defects (which are detected either by a blood test (AFP, see pp76–77) at 15–18 weeks or by a scan).

If you are a carrier of a specific genetic disorder (such as cystic fibrosis), the tissue taken at CVS can often be tested to see whether your baby has the gene that causes the disorder.

Researchers are now developing "panels" of tests that screen for large numbers of genetic defects at one time. Some of these tests may be available in your area for an additional cost or as part of a research protocol, but they are not common.

MAKING THE DECISION

There are several issues to think about before you decide to have CVS. One of the main advantages of CVS is that it can be carried out up to 5 weeks earlier than amniocentesis; this allows for safer, less expensive, and more private pregnancy termination for women who choose this option when an abnormality is found.

In addition, because more genetic material is collected after CVS, the results may be available more quickly than after amniocentesis (about a week or 10 days with CVS; 2 weeks with an amnio). If you are worried about the idea of a needle being inserted into your abdomen (as used when you have an amniocentesis), you may be able to have transcervical CVS, which means there's no need for a needle.

The downside of CVS is that you have to consider the small, but nonetheless real, risk of losing your baby. Here, the experience of the person doing the procedure is important. In skilled hands, the risk of miscarriage after CVS is about 1 in 100 to 1 in 300. This risk is slightly higher than the risk of miscarriage after amniocentesis (1 in 200 to 1 in 400). The rate of

---

RESULTS

■ **What will they tell me about the baby's health?**

The test will tell you whether or not you baby has any chromosomal abnormalities such as Down syndrome, or trisomy 18 or 13. A sample taken at CVS can be used to detect certain single gene disorders such as cystic fibrosis.

■ **What else may the results show?**

Your test may also tell you whether you are having a boy or girl, if you want to know.

■ **How long will my results take?**

The results of the CVS are usually available in 7–10 days.

miscarriage after transabdominal CVS is not different from transcervical CVS. Several years ago, reports suggested a slight risk that the baby might be born with limb abnormalities, including missing fingers or toes. However, most of these cases occurred following CVS that was done before 10 weeks; for this reason, most centres that perform this test will not do CVS earlier than 10 weeks. To put the risk into context, the normal chance of having a baby with a limb defect is around 1 in 1,700. With CVS, this risk may be slightly increased to approximately 1 in 1,000.

Having the Test

Chorionic villus sampling is done in an outpatient clinic. Expect your entire visit to last 1–2 hours, including genetic counselling, the ultrasound, and the procedure.

For you The test is performed using ultrasound guidance so that the doctor can see exactly where the placenta is located. The procedure can be done either through the abdomen (transabdominal) or through the vagina and cervix (transcervical). In the transabdominal procedure, the needle used to collect placental tissue is

Set of chromosomes from a baby with Down syndrome shows an extra number 21 chromosome. Normally each cell has 23 pairs of chromosomes.

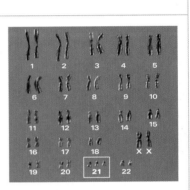

inserted through your abdominal wall. In the transcervical procedure, a slender tube is inserted through the opening of your cervix. Usually, the doctor will decide which approach he or she will take, based on the position of the placenta and the way the doctor was trained. In about 2–3 per cent of cases, the doctor will not be able to perform the procedure because of the position of

the placenta. If this is the case, you have the option of an amniocentesis at 15 weeks. CVS is not very painful for most women. You may have cramps similar to menstrual cramps. If you are having a transabdominal CVS, the needle usually doesn't hurt any more than it does when you have blood taken. Some doctors use a little local anaesthetic before the transabdominal procedure. If your blood type is Rhesus negative you will be given anti-D immune globulin afterwards to prevent complications during this and future pregnancies.

For your baby The CVS procedure collects a sample of placenta – the needle should not touch your baby. The procedure is ultrasound guided and the doctor knows where the needle is at all times. Your baby will not feel any discomfort during the procedure.

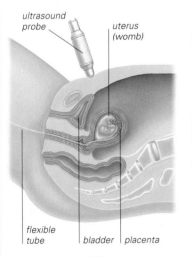

In transcervical CVS, placental tissue is removed through a thin tube passed through the cervix and into the uterus.

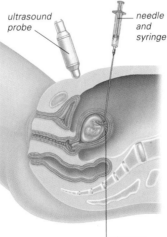

Transabdominal CVS uses a needle inserted through the abdominal wall to collect placental tissue.

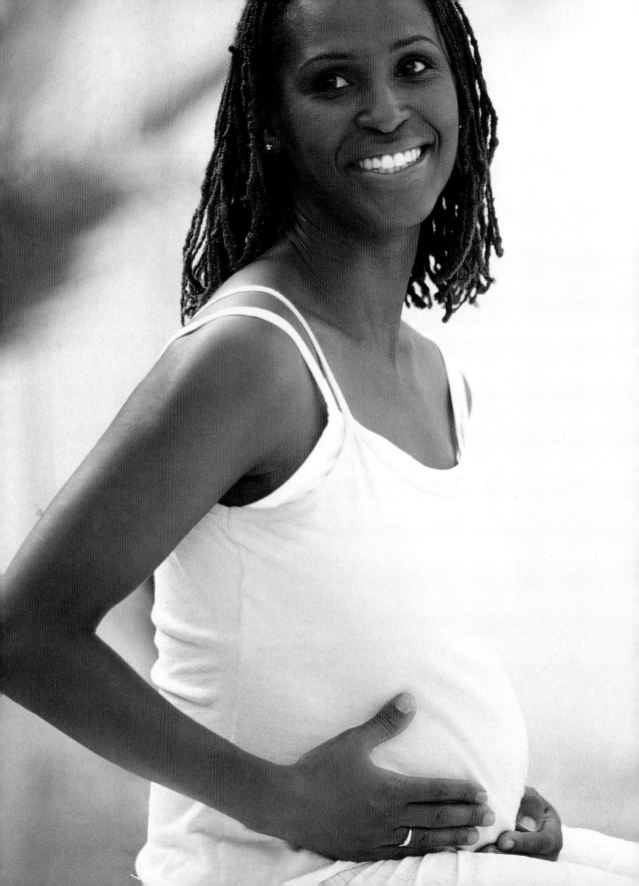

2ND TRIMESTER
what to expect

This trimester is marked by a surge of energy and, for most women, the end of nausea. Your bump will begin to grow and you will start to look obviously pregnant. For many women, these months are the best of all.

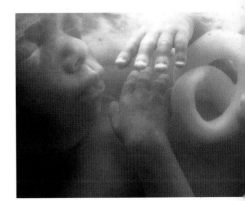

This five-month-old fetus appears fully developed, with perfect facial features and tiny fingers. The umbilical cord can be seen coiled on top of his tummy.

HOW YOU FEEL

You and your partner will be able to share good times together again, and do things you didn't feel like doing in the first 3 months. As your appetite returns and your energy levels rise you may also feel able to enjoy time with friends and family.

Your normal clothes will start to feel tight and while some women avoid maternity clothes for as long as possible, you may find that you have little choice as you get bigger.

At work, you'll probably have the drive to catch up on the things that fell behind during the last months and to plan and work ahead. You may feel you have enough energy to get lots done and are not ready to slow down. The chances you may have a complication that will require you to take sickness leave are slight. However, it may be a good idea to have your job well-organized and be ready to transfer responsibility in case it's necessary in the second half of this trimester. This is especially true for women carrying twins or triplets.

This trimester is a good time to keep active and you are likely to have enough energy for good walks and evenings dancing.

The second trimester is also the time when you might wonder more often about the health of your baby as you wait for the results from tests such as maternal serum screening and amniocentesis.

YOUR BABY

By the start of this trimester your baby will be well-formed. During this period, he or she will grow rapidly, and you will become more aware of each other; your baby's movements will become strong enough for you to feel them. Your baby begins to breathe amniotic fluid in and out, helping to expand and develop the lungs. Amniotic fluid is excreted in the form of urine. By the end of this trimester, your baby's hearing will have developed enough to hear music and the basic elements of your voice. The external genitals will be formed and you may be told the baby's gender at an ultrasound scan.

As your **energy levels rise**, you can **enjoy** spending more time with friends, family, and **your partner**.

your body

By now, the hormonal changes you experienced earlier in your pregnancy will have stabilized, and you should notice your exhaustion and nausea starting to resolve. Breast enlargement, shortness of breath, and dietary cravings will probably continue. During this trimester, your uterus grows to the point where the top will reach your belly button by about 20 weeks.

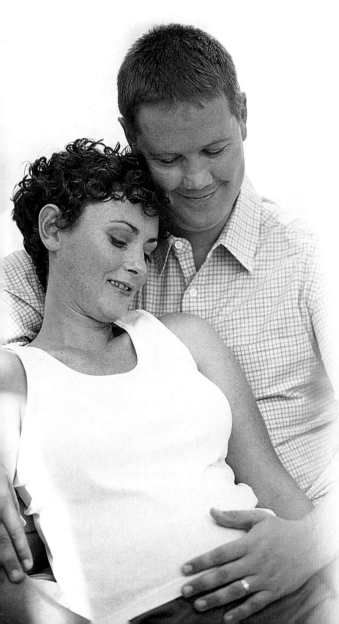

HOW YOUR BODY CHANGES

While your breasts continue to enlarge in preparation for feeding your baby, you can expect that some of the breast tenderness you experienced in the first trimester will resolve. You may feel more open to having your partner touch your breasts during this middle three months of pregnancy.

Your appetite is likely to be at its most intense because your uterus is not yet pressuring your stomach and chest. Any nausea that prevented you from gaining much weight in the first trimester is probably resolving. Expect weight gain not only in your abdomen, but in other areas you may not be as happy about, such as your thighs and hips.

If you have not felt up to exercising in the first trimester, the second trimester is the perfect time to start or renew your fitness regimen (see pp70–71). Keep any activity low impact to protect your softening ligaments and looser joints.

Common problems Towards the end of the second trimester, as the size of your uterus increases, you may notice increasing discomfort. A common cause of second trimester pain is stretching of the ligaments around your uterus, called "round ligament pain". As the weight you carry increases, the risk of back pain also goes up. Since back pain is more common as we age, women over 35 should take extra care to

The excitement of feeling your baby move can be shared with your partner in this trimester. Most women start to feel the baby by around 20 weeks of pregnancy.

What is a Healthy Weight Gain?

Your weight gain may be monitored through your pregnancy. The guidelines on how much weight you should gain in pregnancy are as follows:

Women with a normal pre-pregnancy weight should put on 25–35lb (11–16kg); 35lb (16kg) if having twins. Women who were underweight should gain 28–40lb (13–18kg); women who were overweight before pregnancy should aim to gain up to 15–25lb (7–11kg).

protect their backs from strain. Problems with incontinence (involuntary loss of urine) often begin in the second trimester and are more common in women over 35 (see p103).

FEELING YOUR BABY MOVE

The first time you feel your baby move is an incredible experience. This moment is the beginning of a direct and tangible emotional connection between the two of you.

When will you feel your baby? The stage at which you first feel your baby move depends on several factors – experience, body weight, and position of your placenta. Women who have been pregnant

If you have already had at least one baby, are thin, and your placenta is at the back of the uterus, you may feel your baby move as early as 14–16 weeks. If you are a first-time mum with an anterior placenta and/or you are a bit heavy, you may not feel your baby move until 22–24 weeks. Your care provider will probably ask you if you feel your baby move between 18 and 20 weeks. If you have not felt movement don't get anxious; it doesn't mean there is anything wrong. Most women will have an ultrasound between 20 and 22 weeks gestation, which should reassure you that your baby is moving even if you can't feel it yet.

ONGOING NAUSEA

While most women are rid of pregnancy nausea by the end of the first trimester, some women continue to be nauseated throughout their pregnancy. If you had significant nausea in the first trimester, there is a 25 per cent chance that you will still have some nausea at 20 weeks. However, you can expect that your nausea will slowly decrease as your pregnancy progresses. Only a small percentage of women have nausea that lasts the whole pregnancy. As well as medication (see p39), there are several things you can do to decrease your chances of persistent nausea. Some women's nausea is a result of acid reflux, which gets worse through pregnancy. If your nausea follows

if you've been pregnant before, you're likely to feel your baby move earlier than first-time mums

before usually feel their babies move 1–2 weeks earlier than first-time mums. If the placenta lies along the front of the uterus (anterior position), it acts like a cushion between your skin and your baby and you are less likely to feel your baby move early in your pregnancy. Body weight influences how early you feel movement because subcutaneous fat acts like insulation between you and your baby, and you are less likely to feel your baby move early.

a burning or painful sensation in your chest or is accompanied by a lot of burping, then treatment with antacids may help.

Finally, by this time in your pregnancy you will have identified certain smells or food that trigger nausea. By avoiding these trigger factors you may be able to prevent much of your nausea. Wearing loose clothing can help to reduce the nausea that often results from increased pressure on the abdomen.

your emotions

The second trimester brings many welcome changes. As hormone levels stabilize, you feel more like yourself again. Your energy level is increasing and morning sickness usually fades after the first 12 weeks of pregnancy. Your emotions become more predictable again and your outlook more positive. Being pregnant usually becomes more enjoyable during the second trimester.

FEELING YOUR BABY MOVE

Most women begin to feel their baby move at some point during the second trimester. To begin with, the feeling is very faint and you may not notice it, especially if you are busy or distracted. As your baby grows, the movements become more obvious, and you may begin to notice a connection between your activities and your baby's movements. Many mums are deeply touched when they experience their baby moving for the first time. The feeling makes it clear that there really is another person inside you, and this might make you acknowledge your baby as a new individual in your life for the first time.

If you feel the inclination, spend some time focusing on your baby. A good time is at night, right after you go to bed, since your baby might take a few more minutes than you to wind down, offering you a good opportunity to feel his or her movements and to consciously connect with him or her. For you, this could be the start of the bonding process, and it may be particularly helpful if you have had mixed feelings about becoming a parent.

DEALING WITH UNWANTED ATTENTION

In this trimester it becomes obvious that you are pregnant because your bump becomes visible. Many women do not anticipate how many people will be drawn to touch their stomach uninvited, even strangers. Each individual has her own comfort level with this. Some women enjoy the physical attention. However, if you don't enjoy this type of physical contact, it is okay to set limits; it's not rude to ask

strangers to remove their hands from your body. It is no more appropriate for people, men or women, to touch you without your permission when you are pregnant than when you are not. Don't feel shy about setting boundaries to your personal space. Practise a phrase that you feel at ease with, such as: "I know the urge can be irresistible, but I don't feel comfortable when people touch my stomach." And don't apologize for feeling this way.

During this stage you may also find that you are the recipient of unsolicited advice from all quarters – strangers, your mother, mother-in-law, co-workers, neighbours, and so on. Often, those offering the

> feeling your baby move for the first time is **amazing**, and often **very emotional**

advice may not be up-to-date on the most recent research, but instead offer the conventional wisdom that was accepted when they themselves were pregnant. The advice may be contrary to what you believe, and just plain wrong.

Try hard to filter out unsolicited advice that conflicts with common sense. Remember that this is *your* pregnancy – what is right for you and your baby is up to you and your partner. If you find anything that is said to you interesting or troubling, make a note to discuss it with your doctor or midwife.

ANXIETY OVER TEST RESULTS

More medical tests may be offered to pregnant women who are over 35 than to younger mums, and there is an increased risk of complications for women in this age group and their babies. This fact can make it easy to forget that the vast majority of women over 35 have problem-free pregnancies and healthy babies. Unless there are specific medical problems that warrant greater concern, you are best advised to assume that both you and your baby are perfectly healthy.

If you find your anxiety about tests and their results gets the better of you, acknowledging your fears can help you take charge of them. Gathering medical information, especially about the specific tests, may help to reduce your anxiety. Give your midwife an opportunity to explain what each test does, why it may be necessary, whether there are other options, and how reliable each test is. A good midwife will welcome patients who are actively involved in their own care, so make sure you are in the hands of a competent, supportive team. Gather the down-to-earth facts about the pertinent medical problem. Your local library is a great source of reliable information, as is the internet.

Being worried about unfavourable test results is normal. After all, your life can change dramatically if you or your baby are found to have serious health issues. It might help to consider your options and think about what you would want to do should the outcome of a test prove to be unfavourable, and discuss this with your partner. For some women, believing they are prepared for the worst helps them feel more in control of the situation. Remember, no matter how many or few tests are done, waiting for test results can be unnerving for anyone, but many more times than not there is nothing to worry about.

Getting support Simply voicing your fears can be enough to unravel anxiety and give you a realistic perspective. Talk to your partner, family members, or girlfriends who have been through pregnancy, especially if they were also over 35. A little support while you wait for test results can make waiting much easier.

Your Maternity Wardrobe

During this trimester, your regular clothes stop being comfortable, and you will have to invest in some maternity wear. Some women love pregnancy clothes, while others loathe the idea of switching to the "mummy look", because many maternity clothes are less than stylish and sometimes downright frumpy! Looking good in pregnancy can really raise your spirits and help you feel confident as you adjust to the many changes in your life, so shop thoughtfully for your maternity wardrobe. The following tips may help:

■ When trying maternity clothes, remember that you are likely to grow a lot by the end of your pregnancy, and the gain might not be confined entirely to your stomach.

■ Take into account that seasons may change during your pregnancy, and shop accordingly.

■ If your finances are limited, invest in a few high-quality basics and hunt for more pieces in charity shops, where you can find many barely used bargains. Many women give away their maternity clothes after pregnancy, so ask friends for hand-me-downs. If your job requires you to wear suits or other expensive items, network with other professional women – borrowed maternity clothes can be a fantastic money-saver for a group of sharers.

■ A few dark-coloured skirts and trousers in various fabrics, a good pair of maternity jeans, and two or three comfortable shirts and t-shirts comprise a valuable basic collection.

■ You may sweat more during pregnancy, so buy machine-washable fabrics, especially if you are relying on a limited wardrobe.

your relationships

During the physically easy months of the second trimester, the relationship with your partner may feel much more carefree again and being parents-to-be may become an enjoyable part of your lives. With your energy returning, you will also be able to engage in more activities and catch up with your friends.

SPENDING MORE TIME WITH YOUR PARTNER
Life as a couple now normalizes. Returning energy and waning morning sickness help to dissipate the stress of the early months. Take advantage of this phase – plan time together and recapture the romance in your relationship. If this is your first child, remember that the birth of your baby will change your lives forever, so savour the end of this era as you prepare for the next, and make the most of the time you have together.

Talking to Your Children

After the distractions of the last trimester, you may need to spend special time with your children. Young children need to feel that you are well again and be reassured that they did not cause your earlier distress. This trimester is also a good time to tell them that a new baby is on the way.

Encouraging your child to feel the baby move allows him or her to feel important and included in this exciting family expansion. Young children want to know that they will not be replaced by a new baby, but that they will become the baby's more knowledgeable older sibling. Encourage them to feel this way by explaining all the good things about being a big brother or sister.

Older children also benefit from time spent with you in harmony after the difficult first trimester. As your pregnancy advances, they may be embarrassed that everyone can see that their parents are sexually active. They may also be afraid they will become perpetual babysitters.

Encourage your child to discuss his or her feelings about the expected arrival, and do all you can to prepare your child for the big change ahead.

Sex It's back and it's more fun than ever! The physical changes of pregnancy go beyond your growing belly and several can make your sex life more pleasurable than ever before. Your breasts enlarge and your nipples darken – your partner may enjoy these changes particularly. Your nipples also become more sensitive so that your partner's touch is even more pleasing to you. In addition, your labia and clitoris swell slightly and are more easily excitable.

preparing for your baby's arrival together is **exciting.** It's the first thing you do **together as parents**

Women often feel intensely aroused and reach their climax more quickly while they are pregnant. For their partners, this enhanced sensitivity and the resulting vaginal lubrication makes penetration an especially sensual experience.

Feeling unattractive Some women find it difficult to adjust to their expanding waistlines and feel unattractive in maternity clothes. Some men may wonder, too, whether they will find their partners attractive during pregnancy. Try and enjoy your increased voluptuousness. Remember that pregnancy is highly feminine, and many men find pregnancy very arousing. Your confidence in your own sexuality will go a long way to exciting your partner.

With so many new possibilities for sexual pleasure during this trimester, it would be a pity for you to focus on any negative feelings you may have about yourself. Try to relax and enjoy intimacy. Use this time to heal some of the bruises that a possibly long and arduous preconception time and an exhausting first trimester may have left in your love life. Forget about your waistline, take off your maternity clothes, and focus on your exciting sexual assets.

LOOKING FORWARD TO BEING PARENTS

During this trimester, your pregnancy will become a certain reality. You will receive your test results and will most likely find that your baby is developing well. You will also feel the first movements of your child. At this point, you might finally feel free to look forward whole-heartedly to becoming a parent and to make plans for your baby. The pregnancy also becomes very real for your partner when he begins to feel the baby kick. This is a big moment for him.

Now is a good time to plan for your baby, since you can expect your energy level to decrease again in the last trimester, and your days will quickly fill with frequent medical check-ups and preparations for leaving work. You could consider names for your baby, plan his or her nursery, and shop for the first baby items. Sometimes grandparents will have heirloom baby furniture that needs to be fixed up for your baby. Now is a good time for such time-consuming, work-intensive projects. Any that involve substances such as paint thinners and strippers or paint,

Take advantage of boosted energy
to catch up with friends and socialize
in this relatively calm trimester.

which could be dangerous to your baby, are ideal projects for your partner. Planning and preparing for your child together will help your partner feel involved.

SPENDING TIME WITH FRIENDS

Your boosted energy level may also allow you to spend more time with your friends and extended family again. This may be a good time for you to tell them about your pregnancy. Many of these relationships will change with the arrival of your baby. Take advantage, therefore, of the opportunity to socialize.

You might find that your relationships with women friends who have children begin to take on added dimensions because there is more that you can share. It is helpful for you to have someone with whom you can share your excitement and your fears. Receiving advice and observing other mums with their children can help you feel more at ease with motherhood.

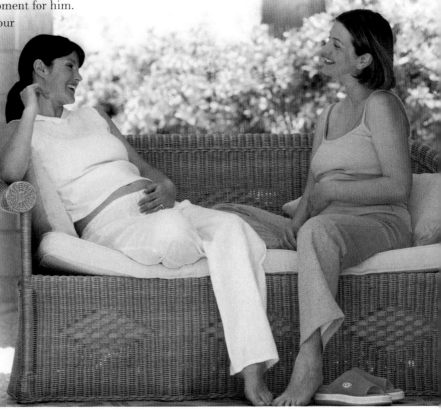

your career

Working in the second trimester is, for many women, the most comfortable period of working while pregnant. The intense loss of energy during the first trimester is diminishing, and you may feel more inclined to tackle some of the bigger challenges in your work life. You could reap the rewards of this when you return to work, but make sure you don't deplete your energy.

CONSERVING YOUR ENERGY

After the intense fatigue of the first trimester, you may feel a sense of great liberation, now that it's easier to move and even think again. You may be tempted to add to your schedule all those things you had eliminated at the beginning of your pregnancy.

Within reason, take advantage of your current boost in energy – working hard now will help to win favour with your employers, which could make it easier for them to be flexible with you when you need using your keyboard. A screen guard can also help reduce glare from monitors and may stop or reduce eye fatigue. If you are on your feet a lot in your job, take regular rests, and enquire about whether or not you can spend more time sitting down. Be sure to wear comfortable clothes and shoes.

Travel If your job requires a good deal of travel, you'll find this is easiest in the second trimester of pregnancy, especially between 18 and 24 weeks

planning for your maternity leave, or for your life after you leave work, can be very exciting

to slow down in the third trimester, or when you return to work. Although you have more energy, be careful to pay attention to your body's signals and not overdo it. This isn't good for your baby and you may need even longer to recover later. Increase your commitments with caution, and don't over-exert yourself. Prioritize tasks, doing important ones first.

CONSIDERING COMFORT

Do all you can to ensure your comfort at work. For example, make sure your chair gives your back the support you need, and that your work station is set up correctly. If you use a computer, check that your chair is the correct height in relation to your monitor in order to avoid neck and back pain. Try using a wrist rest to see if it makes you feel more comfortable when the risk of any pregnancy complications developing is at its lowest.

It is essential that you drink enough water to prevent dehydration, which can decrease blood flow to your baby and put you at risk of developing deep vein thrombosis (blood clots) in your legs. Take regular breaks from your seat to stretch your legs. Don't allow travelling to put strain on your bladder. If you are driving, stop regularly to empty your bladder, and empty your bladder right before getting on a plane.

To ensure at least minimal comfort when travelling by air, ask for a seat with more legroom when you make your reservation and for an extra pillow to support your back during your flight. Don't worry about the X-rays at security check-points. They are not harmful to your baby.

PLANNING YOUR MATERNITY LEAVE

Some women choose to become full-time mums after the birth of their babies. For others this is financially impossible, undesirable, or both. If you plan to return to work, you'll have to think about maternity leave. In the UK, pregnant employees are entitled to 26 weeks' ordinary maternity leave (see p15).

Timing your departure Many women stay at work as long as possible so they can spend most of their leave with their babies. This also allows time for unexpected medical problems that might arise after the birth. As part of your planning, you need to seriously consider how you would manage if you were placed on bedrest during the second half of pregnancy. Bedrest is more common in women over 35 due to the increased risk of high blood pressure. Consider whether you would continue to work from home, or if you would have to go on maternity leave early (see p90). Balance your personal needs and work commitments to establish a sensible time for you to begin your leave.

CHOOSING TO LEAVE WORK

Leaving work permanently after you become pregnant is a life-changing decision. For some women, this has always been the plan. If this describes you, your choice is likely to be the result of planning and reflects your values, so leaving work will be right for you.

Points to consider If you are for the first time considering leaving work, bear in mind the following factors. You will lose the companionship of your associates, the financial security and freedom that your income provides, and the regularity of a daily routine. If you get a strong sense of identity from your career role, this will also be lost. Furthermore, being a full-time mum might not suit you, and you may be happier in the long term if you continue to work, part-time if not full-time. If possible, wait until you are on maternity leave to make the final decision so you can try out life at home with a baby 24 hours a day. You may find it is not what you expected.

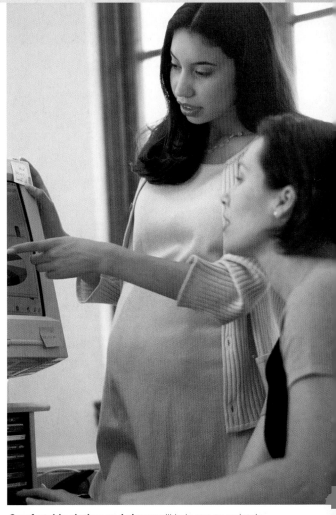

Comfortable clothes and shoes will help you to maintain your concentration at work as well as your energy. A sensible maternity wardrobe is well worth the cost.

It's your decision Sometimes, the decision to leave or stay at work is due to pressure from other people. Some men encourage their pregnant partners to give up work so that they themselves can concentrate fully on their own careers without making compromises because of childcare considerations. Similarly, some women who would rather stay at home with their children feel they must return to work for financial reasons since their partner has a fun but poorly paid job that he is unwilling to give up. Make sure this is your own choice and that you've made it rationally.

exercise programme

Often, it is not until after nausea and fatigue have diminished that you can consider beginning an exercise programme or continuing your pre-pregnancy routine. Nausea tends to recede in the second trimester and, for many women, this trimester is the least tiring one. Now is the ideal time to exercise.

RECOMMENDED EXERCISES

Choose aerobic activities with minimal risk of injury, such as walking or stationary cycling, and stick to your target heart rate (see p47). Limit your exercise to moderate intensity. As your baby grows, you'll feel him or her move during and right after exercise. Babies tend to have favourite activities, so plan for more of those activities that your baby enjoys!

YOUR SAFETY

You may feel much more energetic again during the second trimester, but remember that physical activity is hard on your body, and excessive exercise can harm your baby. When you exercise, your needs are met before your baby's. Blood flow is diverted to the muscles that do most of the work, which can decrease the blood supply available for your baby. When you exercise at a high intensity (when you feel that you are working out "very hard"), your baby may not receive a healthy amount of blood. Exercising at a moderate rate (a rate that feels "somewhat hard") is fine.

Keeping your balance Your centre of gravity shifts during pregnancy and you can easily lose your balance, even during familiar exercise moves. To decrease your

IDEAL EXERCISE ACTIVITIES FOR THE 2ND TRIMESTER

	Benefits and suggestions	Frequency and duration
Hiking and brisk walking	Hiking improves cardiovascular health, and doing it in a place of natural beauty will recharge your batteries. A brisk walk during your lunch hour at work is also good exercise, and will refresh you for the afternoon.	Daily if possible, or at least four times a week. Aim for 30 minutes if it feels comfortable.
Stationary cycling	Switching from your outdoor bike to a stationary one (in the comfort of a climate-controlled environment) can prevent serious falls as your balance diminishes. Also, you can track the duration of your workout.	Four or five times a week if this is your only exercise. Up to 30 minutes is fine (45 mins maximum).
Elliptical training	Changing from jogging to working out on an elliptical machine eliminates the stress on your abdominal, lower back, and pelvic floor muscles. This can prevent lower back pain and pelvic floor weakness.	Four to five times per week if this is your only exercise. Up to 30 minutes is fine (45 mins maximum).
Modified abdominal exercises	Avoid traditional abdominal crunches. Try lying on your side to crunch, or get on your hands and knees and make a cat back. Use an exercise ball for gentle but deep abdominal exercises that are safe in pregnancy.	Do three sets of 8–10 repetitions at least twice a week (no more than three times a week).

risk of injury, avoid activities requiring good balance, particularly towards the end of your second trimester.

Keep cool Exercising outdoors in hot weather or relaxing in a hot tub can raise your body temperature to 39°C (102°F), which may be detrimental to the development of your baby's central nervous system. You may want to schedule outdoor activities for cooler morning or evening hours during summer and wear exercise clothing appropriate for the season. Or you may prefer to exercise in air-conditioned indoor facilities during summer.

Unfortunately, your after-exercise relaxation in a hot tub should be eliminated from your activity list atogether while you are pregnant.

Avoid environmental pollution Exercising in high traffic areas can increase the amount of lead you breathe to harmful levels for your baby. Avoid unclean swimming pools – they may increase your risk of urinary tract or yeast infection and add to the regular discomforts of pregnancy.

Avoid lying on your back Lying flat on your back decreases the blood volume pumped by your heart by 9 per cent, probably because your baby's weight prevents blood flow from your legs back to your heart. Turning on your side during exercise prevents this problem.

Benefits of Moderate Exercise

Exercising regularly in the second trimester can help alleviate or avoid several common (and less common) pregnancy complaints.

Injury prevention As your centre of gravity shifts and your ligaments relax, you are more prone to problems with balance and injury. Continued strength training can alleviate this problem.

Improved body image The many medical tests of early pregnancy, fatigue, and nausea can make you feel like a sick patient. Exercise helps you feel confident in your body's ability to support a healthy pregnancy.

Controlled weight gain Exercise helps you gain less fat and gain weight within recommended limits.

*An **exercise ball** allows for some gentle abdominal exercises during pregnancy, and can double up as a labour prop.*

food plan

For many women, this trimester brings welcome relief from morning sickness, and you will probably start to enjoy food again. If the change does not come with the first days of the second trimester, be patient. You may see a gradual improvement over the next few weeks.

Once you can enjoy food again, it's time to focus on a diet that meets your nutritional needs. A balanced diet reliant on fresh produce supplies a broad range of nutrients that will support your baby's development and your wellbeing.

Your vitamin and mineral requirements are generally higher in pregnancy than before although you need to be sure to avoid megadoses, especially of vitamins A and D (see p48). In this trimester it's worth rechecking your intake.

Sources of Vitamin C

Your vitamin C requirements double in pregnancy. The best sources for this vitamin are as follows.

- Citrus fruits and berries such as raspberries and strawberries.
- Citrus fruit juices such as orange and grapefruit juice (one glass of fortified orange juice supplies all the vitamin C you need for a day).
- Papaya, guava, and kiwifruit.
- Green leafy vegetables such as cauliflower, broccoli, cabbage, and spinach.

YOUR NUTRITIONAL NEEDS

Laying the foundations for healthy weight gain in you and your baby now will give your baby the best start in life. It will also benefit your health throughout your pregnancy and after delivery.

Eating for two You need to eat more while your body supports the growth of your baby, but not twice as much as before pregnancy. Only 300 extra calories per day are needed throughout pregnancy to ensure optimal growth of your baby. All extra calories will be stored by your body as fat.

Just two to four extra servings per day cover your increased energy needs. For instance, 100g (4oz) of low-fat cottage cheese has 90 calories, and 100g (4oz) of skinless chicken breast has 140. Take into account that you may be snacking throughout the day. A small handful of peanuts supplies 160 calories. Energy bars can contain 160–300 calories.

It's easy to overestimate the amount of extra food you need. Therefore, find out the caloric content of your favourite foods and snacks, and the number of

servings that cover your additional needs. Only 2–4kg (5–9lb) of the weight you gain during pregnancy is typically body weight gain. The rest is accounted for by the weight of your baby and his or her support system (amniotic fluid, a larger uterus and placenta, and larger breasts in preparation for the arrival of your baby).

The average increase in weight may be 1–2kg (2–4lb) during the first trimester, 5.5–6kg (12–14lb) during the second, and 3.5–4.5kg (8–10lb) in the last.

Gaining enough weight during your pregnancy decreases your risk of delivering a low birth-weight baby – a baby that weighs less than 2.5kg (5.5lb). However, gaining too much weight may leave you at risk of developing gestational diabetes (see p110) and of having a large baby. Excess weight gain often causes women to remain overweight after the birth, and the older you are, the harder it is to shift this excess weight.

Vitamin C The recommended daily allowance of vitamin C for pregnant women is 70mg – twice as much as in nonpregnant women.

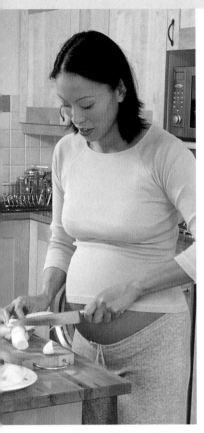

Your well-balanced diet should include plenty of fresh produce. Avoid pre-prepared meals whenever possible.

Some of this can be obtained from antenatal vitamins but you should still have enough in your diet. Vitamin C promotes the absorption of iron and calcium, both of which are important for you and your baby, and is also important in many processes in the body. The best sources for vitamin C are fruits and vegetables (see opposite).

FOOD CRAVINGS

Many women experience cravings during pregnancy. Chocolate and other sweets, ice cream, spicy foods, fruit, and fish rank at the top of the list of must-haves, often in unusual combinations.

No one knows why women have cravings. Experts have varying opinions. Some say that cravings are psychological – part of our culture. They believe women learn to expect cravings and consequently have them. Some researchers feel hormonal changes in pregnancy, especially increased progesterone, cause cravings. Similar cravings in menopausal women support this opinion. It does not explain the variety in foods craved, however. Some propose that hunger for a certain food indicates a woman's need for nutrients in that food. This may be true, but is questionable with cravings for sweets, which contain little more than sugar.

Yet another explanation is that emotional factors contribute to cravings. Pregnancy greatly impacts on your life and indulging in a craving is emotionally gratifying, especially if your partner shows his devotion by hunting for the impossible food combination of your choice at midnight.

The reality is that nobody knows what causes food cravings. Most women would insist they are real and can be overwhelming at times. The most probable explanation may be a complex interplay of physical changes, learned behaviour, and emotional needs.

Dealing with food cravings

Indulging your cravings for certain foods can make you feel better, physically and emotionally. But if the foods you crave are high in calories, harmful fats, and sugar, set healthy limits for yourself. Taking charge of your cravings is not difficult. Try the following strategies to help you control them.

- Substitute the food you crave with healthier choices, at least some of the time. For example, have non-fat frozen yogurt instead of ice cream.
- Eat breakfast every day. There's some evidence that skipping breakfast increases cravings.
- Exercise regularly. Physical activity controls your appetite by elevating blood sugar levels. Exercise also takes you away from your kitchen and your thoughts away from your craving.
- Make sure you have emotional support. Pregnancy taxes your emotional resources, especially if you are juggling a changing relationship with your partner, a career, and a full social life. This may cause you to reach for some comfort food when in fact all you need is a hug.

Unusual cravings Some women begin to crave non-food items such as ice, dirt, paint, coffee grounds, chalk, cornflour, cigarette ashes, soap, and toothpaste. This is known as pica and, even though none of the listed items contains iron, pica has been associated with iron deficiency. If you experience pica, you should inform your healthcare provider right away. Non-food items may contain toxic substances that may be harmful to your baby.

antenatal care

Thankfully, complications in the second trimester of pregnancy are rare.
Because of this, unless you have a medical condition that needs monitoring, you
will generally see your care provider infrequently during this period. However,
because visits are few and far between, it makes sense to know the signs of
potential problems, such as preterm labour, that should prompt you to call in.

At each antenatal visit during this trimester (about every 4–6 weeks) your doctor or midwife will check your blood pressure. You will also be asked to give a urine sample, which is checked for protein and sugar. Protein is rarely found at this point in your pregnancy, but if it is it may be a sign of preeclampsia (see p113). Sugar in the urine can be a sign of gestational diabetes (see p110).

At every visit after 12 weeks, you can expect to hear your baby's heartbeat with a device called a Doppler (sonicaid). After 20 weeks your healthcare provider may start to measure the size of your uterus with a tape measure to check your baby's growth. During the early part of this trimester, you will be given the option of tests to check for Down syndrome or other chromosome abnormalities (see below). If you have had first trimester testing or chorionic villus sampling (CVS), your care provider should offer you isolated testing for neural tube defects (spina bifida) using the blood test for alpha-fetoprotein (AFP) or an ultrasound scan. Most care providers will order an ultrasound between 18 and 21 weeks to make sure your baby is well-formed.

CALLING YOUR DOCTOR

Although most women will have a normal, healthy second trimester, you should be aware of situations in which you need to call your healthcare provider immediately.

SECOND TRIMESTER TESTS

Name of test	What the results show	How the test is done
Amniocentesis (see p80–81)	Definitive diagnosis of Down syndrome, trisomy 18, and other chromosomal abnormalities.	Sample of amniotic fluid is removed using a needle guided by ultrasound. Cells from the sample are cultured and chromosomes are analysed under a microscope. Commonly done at 15–18 weeks.
Maternal serum screening (see p76–77)	Estimated risk of Down syndrome or trisomy 18.	Blood sample is taken and tested for three (triple test) or four (quad test) body chemicals. The risk of Down syndrome or trisomy 18 is calculated by combining these results with age and due date. Test is done at 15–18 weeks.
Ultrasound (see p78–79)	Detects various abnormalities, including neural tube defects and heart abnormalities.	Detailed ultrasound scan is performed by experienced doctor or sonographer. The ultrasound probe is moved over the tummy to view the fetus in the uterus. The scan is usually done at 18–21 weeks.

Vaginal bleeding Any vaginal bleeding should prompt you to call the hospital. Most vaginal bleeding in pregnancy comes from the cervix and is not usually serious. Vaginal spotting often occurs after intercourse because the cervix has a lot of fragile blood vessels on the surface. This does not mean that intercourse is harmful. Any vaginal bleeding more than spotting should prompt an immediate call to your obstetric care provider. You may have a placenta praevia (where the placenta has implanted over the cervical opening) or placental abruption (where the edge of the placenta has started to peel away from the wall of the uterus). If you are more than 24 weeks pregnant and you have any bright red bleeding that soaks your underwear, call your doctor or go to hospital immediately.

Increased vaginal discharge
Vaginal discharge often increases with pregnancy. However, if you notice a sudden and abrupt increase in your discharge, and especially if it is thin and mucousy, you should call your doctor. In some cases, increased discharge results from your cervix opening up (called cervical insufficiency, see p111).

Sudden vaginal pressure As your baby grows, a gradual increase in pressure is normal. However, if you feel sudden vaginal pressure, or have the

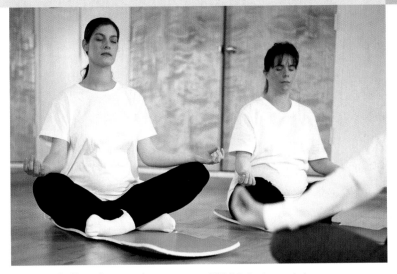

Childbirth classes help you prepare for labour. Some classes use yoga techniques to teach relaxation.

constant feeling that you have to have a bowel movement, call the hospital at once because this may be a sign of preterm labour.

Gush of clear fluid If you have a large gush of clear fluid that soaks your clothes call the hospital immediately; sometimes this is a symptom of the amniotic sac breaking. While urinary incontinence increases during pregnancy, you should not attribute a gush of fluid to loss of bladder control unless you are absolutely certain this is the case.

Diarrhoea with abdominal pain
If you have diarrhoea with a lot of abdominal pain, you may want to check in with your care provider in case you are in preterm labour.

STARTING CHILDBIRTH CLASSES
In the mid to late second trimester you might start thinking about childbirth classes. Whether you want to take classes or not depends

on how you learn best; they are not compulsory. Some women prefer to read about childbirth and ask their care provider any questions they have. Other women may prefer to learn directly from a labour expert, and have a chance to ask questions face-to-face.

Childbirth classes can be helpful for partners, allowing them to address their anxieties and ask questions. Classes are often offered through the facility where you plan to deliver. Some women prefer an independent class. Such classes are often designed around a particular philosophy of managing labour pain, and the information they provide may be biased against receiving pain medication in labour.

What you choose is a personal decision. The bottom line is that the class fits with your philosophy and still supplies you with factual information about labour.

maternal serum screening

Second trimester serum screening, or maternal serum screening as it is also called, is a simple blood test that will tell whether or not your baby has an increased risk of being affected by Down syndrome, trisomy 18, or neural tube defects (such as spina bifida). As with any other screening test, participation is optional and whether or not you want to be screened is a personal decision.

WHAT IS THE TEST?

The test is based on a blood sample taken at between 15 and 18 weeks of pregnancy. The sample is then tested for either three ("triple screen") or four ("quad screen") blood chemicals. With the triple screen, your blood is tested for three specific substances: alpha-fetoprotein (AFP), human chorionic gonadotropin (hCG), and unconjugated oestriol. With the quad screen, a fourth marker called inhibin A is also included.

Your personal levels of these blood chemicals are combined with your age into a formula that calculates your baby's individual risk of Down syndrome or trisomy 18. Your risk may be higher or lower than your risk would have been based on your age alone, or it may remain the same.

A "positive" or "high-risk" test result does not mean that your baby has Down syndrome, only that your risk is higher than the normal risk in a woman aged 35.

If the test finds you have high AFP levels, it may mean your baby is at higher risk of having a neural tube defect such as spina bifida (see opposite) or other problems. A blood sample can also be tested for AFP alone if you have already had first trimester screening (see pp56–57) or chorionic villus sampling (CVS, see pp58–59),

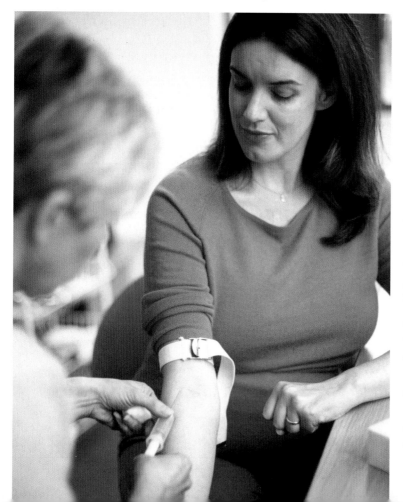

A sample of blood is taken at 15–18 weeks of pregnancy and analysed in the laboratory. From this analysis, the risk of Down syndrome can be calculated.

Neural Tube Defects

One of the chemicals tested in the triple and quad test is alpha-fetoprotein (AFP). A high AFP may indicate that your baby may have neural tube defects (such as spina bifida). Neural tube defects mean that the spine has not formed properly early in development, leaving the spinal cord unprotected and exposed to the amniotic fluid in the uterus. The closer to the head the defect occurs in the spine, the more major problems the baby is likely to have. Affected children can have extra fluid in the brain, leg paralysis, and lack of bladder and bowel control. However, high AFP levels are also present if you are carrying twins or your pregnancy is further along than you thought. If you have a high AFP test, the next step is to have a level II ultrasound (see pp78–79), which is performed by a specialist in detailed ultrasound examinations. About 95 per cent of babies with neural tube defect can be detected by ultrasound.

neither of which detect neural tube defects, although many hospitals just offer a scan.

DECIDING TO BE TESTED

There are several reasons why maternal serum screening might be a good choice for you. Maybe you missed out on first trimester screening, either because the test is not available in your area or your first pregnancy visit was too late. Alternatively, you may have had first trimester screening or CVS, but want screening for neural tube defects, which isn't detected by either of these tests.

However, you need to remember that this blood test, while having the advantage over amniocentesis of posing no risk at all to your baby, isn't infallible. You may be told your risk is low and then still go on to have a baby with Down syndrome. Conversely, you may be told you are at higher risk but have a perfectly normal baby.

Test accuracy In women over the age of 35, second trimester screening will detect more than 80 per cent of babies with Down syndrome but misses 20 per cent of Down syndrome babies. The detection rate depends on whether you have the triple screen or the quad screen and on your age. As a general rule, the quad test is less likely than the triple test to give you a false positive result. If you have the choice, it is the best test to have if you are under 40. However, if you absolutely must know whether your baby has Down syndrome, you should skip this test and move directly to having an amniocentesis.

DEALING WITH THE RESULT

Even if your test is positive, the chance of your baby having Down syndrome is still fairly low. The results should tell you the exact risk of Down syndrome in your pregnancy — you can then compare this risk to the risk of having a miscarriage with amniocentesis. Remember that you do not have to have an amnio just because you have a positive screening test; it's your choice. If your blood test is negative, there is a very low chance of your baby having Down syndrome and you will not be offered an amniocentesis.

RESULTS

■ **What will they tell me about the baby's health?**
The results will only tell you whether there is a high or low risk of your baby having Down syndrome or other chromosomal abnormality. The results may also tell you if your baby is at higher risk for a neural tube defect (see above). Since your pregnancy dating is part of the calculation, the test may be inaccurate if you recall your last menstrual period wrongly. The test is less accurate in twins.

■ **How long will my results take?**
You will normally get your results about a week after having the test. The results are in the form of a report that your doctor will discuss with you.

ultrasound

Most women have an ultrasound at some stage in pregnancy. If you have only one it is likely to be between 18 and 22 weeks. There are three main purposes of an ultrasound examination – to make sure that the size of the baby matches your due date; to look at how the baby is formed; and to evaluate your placenta and amniotic fluid to make sure they are normal.

Ultrasound uses sound waves to produce images of your baby in the uterus. The sound waves are emitted from a probe, and they bounce off your baby and produce an image that can be seen on a monitor. Ultrasound provides your care provider with a lot of information about your baby's development and wellbeing.

HAVING THE SCAN

You'll lie on your back with your abdomen exposed and a gel will be applied to your skin. The doctor or sonographer will then move a probe over your belly and the baby's image will appear on the screen. An ultrasound scan can take 15–20 minutes (for a basic scan) or up to 90 minutes for a level II (detailed) scan. You may have a level II scan if there have been any concerns raised about your baby in an earlier ultrasound or other examination.

YOUR DUE DATE

Your due date is calculated from the date of your last menstrual period. However, the ultrasound

What Ultrasound Shows

Detection of abnormalities, especially subtle ones, is better in centres that specialize in antenatal diagnosis. Most hospitals refer for a level II scan if they suspect that there may be a problem.

■ Size of baby

The baby's head, abdomen, and thigh bone are measured to find the baby's size and check that he or she is the right size for how far along you are.

■ Brain, heart, and other organs

Abnormalities such as extra fluid inside the brain, and major heart defects may be seen. Even if no major structural abnormalities are seen, some findings are important because they slightly increase the chance of Down syndrome. If you have already had CVS or amniocentesis you can be reassured. Otherwise a combination of abnormalities may suggest to the doctors that you should be referred to a fetal medicine centre. Other findings may indicate an increased risk of minor health problems. One example is extra fluid in the kidneys, which could be a sign of a problem with how your baby's kidneys drain. This problem, called urinary reflux, is more common in boys and is readily confirmed after birth and usually resolves over time.

■ Neural tube defects

An ultrasound scan can detect 95 per cent of babies with neural tube defects, such as spina bifida. (See also p77.)

■ Hands, feet, limbs, and facial features

Physical problems such as cleft lip and club foot will usually show up on an ultrasound scan.

■ Placenta and amniotic fluid

Your ultrasound will confirm that your placenta is in the correct place and not blocking the cervix (placenta praevia, see p113). The scan will also check the level of amniotic fluid.

scan is often used to confirm this date. If your ultrasound scan shows your baby to be larger or smaller than would be expected, your due date may be recalculated.

CHECKING YOUR BABY

The ultrasound will look at the fluid inside the baby's brain, the shape of the back of the baby's brain, the spine, the upper lip, the heart, the stomach, the kidneys, the bladder, the arms, legs, hands, and feet. The scan will also look for structural problems with your baby like neural tube defects, cleft lip, club foot, heart defects, and brain abnormalities (see opposite.)

Ultrasound can only look at how your baby is formed, not how particular organs work. The ultrasound will not be able to tell if your baby will have normal intelligence, or if your baby's liver will function properly.

Down syndrome Ultrasound alone is not a good way to rule out Down syndrome. However, it can pick up so-called "soft" signs, which may slightly increase the chance that your baby has Down syndrome. The following may prompt further investigation.

- Short leg or arm bones.
- Absent or short nasal bone.
- Thickened skin at the back of your baby's neck.
- A bright spot seen in your baby's heart (echogenic cardiac focus) slightly increases the risk. However, this finding does not

mean that your baby is more likely to have a heart defect. Most babies with an echogenic cardiac focus have an absolutely normal heart.

- Extra fluid in one or both of your baby's kidneys (called pylectasis). This finding may also be a sign of urinary reflex, which is not serious and often resolves over time after the baby is born (see box, opposite).
- Choroid plexus cysts – tiny bubble-like structures seen in the organ that makes the fluid that surrounds your baby's brain. These are not uncommon, and more than 99 per cent disappear before birth. If your baby's chromosomes are normal, cysts do not mean there is a problem with your baby's intelligence or his or her development.
- Curved littlest finger, which is found in about 1 in 100 normal babies but is more common in Down syndrome babies.

If you have had reassuring first or second trimester screening for Down syndrome, then detecting a single one of these signs on its own is not a cause for concern. However, if you have not had screening, or you have a positive screen and two or more soft markers are seen, the findings will be discussed with you and you may be referred to a fetal medicine centre for a second opinion. While the chance that your baby has Down syndrome is still fairly low, these findings may

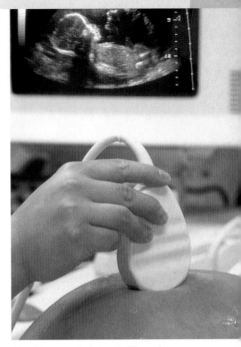

An ultrasound at about 20 weeks *gives a great view of your baby and provides a lot of information about his or her development and wellbeing.*

alter your feelings about amniocentesis or cordocentesis. Some kinds of heart defects are more serious but you will almost certainly be referred for a special heart test to diagnose them correctly first.

BOY OR GIRL?

Unless the baby is curled up or has his or her legs closed tight, you should be able to get a pretty good idea of whether you are having a boy or girl when you have an ultrasound. If you don't want to know the gender of your baby, make sure to tell the sonographer. Some hospitals have a policy of not disclosing the baby's sex, others will tell you if you ask.

amniocentesis

An amniocentesis provides a definite answer to the question of whether or not your baby has a chromosomal problem – such as Down syndrome or trisomy 18 – or a neural tube defect. This test is usually offered to women over 35 because of the increased risk of chromosome abnormalities after this age. The procedure is usually done between 15 and 18 weeks.

In the uterus, your baby is protected and cushioned by amniotic fluid within an amniotic sac. The amniotic fluid mainly consists of your baby's urine together with some cells from his or her skin and urinary tract. With amniocentesis, a sample of this fluid is withdrawn and cells are collected and grown in the lab. When there are enough cells, the chromosomes inside (which carry the genetic material) are then viewed and analysed. This can take up to 3 weeks.

MAKING THE DECISION

Your doctor may discuss the possibility of having an amnio after receiving the results of your first trimester screen including a nuchal fold scan (see pp56–57). Alternatively, you may consider having an amnio because you want to know for certain whether or not your baby has Down syndrome.

There are pros and cons to consider. The results will give you concrete information, but the test carries a small risk of miscarriage.

This risk is around 0.25 to 0.5 per cent (in other words, 1 in 200 to 1 in 400 women will miscarry after an amnio). Some women are so determined to have their baby, regardless of problems, they feel having the test is an unnecessary risk. Others struggle with the idea of a diminished quality of life for their child and want to know for certain what they might have to face. Opting for a test that carries a slim chance of losing the baby is a difficult decision to make. Each couple must decide how important it is to have the information that an amniocentesis provides.

If the test is positive, they then have to consider whether or not to terminate the pregnancy. Your doctor can discuss these issues with you, and you may find talking to close friends, family members, or a counsellor helpful.

LOOKING AFTER YOURSELF

Many women who have had an amnio say it helps to imagine the experience as a three-hurdle process, and to concentrate on one hurdle at a time. First is the test itself; second are the hours after the

---

RESULTS

■ **How long will my results take?**

You may be able to get preliminary results within a few days, if you are willing to pay for extra testing, but these must be confirmed by the main test result, which takes up to 3 weeks.

■ **What will they tell me about the baby's health?**

The final purpose of an amnio is to rule out the possibility that your baby has Down syndrome or another chromosomal abnormality.

■ **What other information can be learned from an amniocentesis?**

An amniocentesis can test for other chromosomal abnormalities, apart from Down syndrome. The procedure may also be used if there is a risk of the baby having a genetic disease such as cystic fibrosis, although this is not done routinely. From an amniocentesis, you can also find out the sex of your baby if you wish to know it.

test, when the risk of miscarriage is greatest; and finally there's the result, which can take up to 3 weeks to arrive. Take someone with you when you go for the test so that you have some support.

WHAT ARE THE RISKS?

The risk of miscarriage following amniocentesis is between 1 in 200 and 1 in 400, and the chances of losing the baby reduce as the hours and days go by after the procedure. If everything is all right 5 days after the test, your chances of losing the baby are slim. Seek help if there is vaginal bleeding, abdominal cramping, or loss of clear fluids.

Having the Test

Amniocentesis is done as an outpatient procedure and takes about 20–40 minutes. (Most of this time is for the ultrasound part of the procedure). After you have had the test, you will be advised to take it easy for the remainder of the day.

For you The test will be carried out by a doctor with the assistance of an experienced medical sonographer who will use ultrasound to get a clear view of your uterus. Your abdomen will be wiped with antiseptic before the doctor inserts a long, thin, hollow needle through it into the amniotic cavity inside your womb, guided by the ultrasound at all times. You may notice some cramping as the needle goes through the wall of the uterus, rather like menstrual cramping. Women who have been through the procedure describe the test as uncomfortable rather than painful. The doctor will almost certainly be willing to explain everything to you and point out what's happening on the screen. Once the amnio is complete, the doctor may monitor you for a minute or so to make sure that the fetus is still well and you can go home safely after the procedure.

For your baby Having a needle inserted into your uterus, near your growing baby, sounds scary, but every precaution is taken to ensure the baby's safety. The ultrasound enables the doctor to find a pocket of amniotic fluid at a safe distance from the baby. As soon as the needle is in place, the sharp point is withdrawn so that even if the baby reaches out and touches the tube he or she will not be harmed.

Amniocentesis does carry some risks for your pregnancy. The chances of miscarriage are higher if there are problems during the procedure itself. If there are no obvious problems, the chances of losing your baby as a result of the procedure are very low.

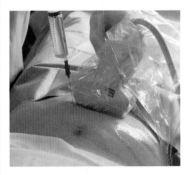

A needle is inserted into your abdomen by a highly skilled doctor. The procedure is not usually painful.

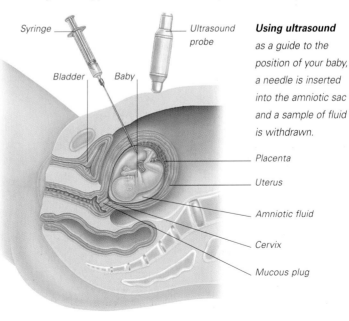

Syringe

Ultrasound probe

Bladder   Baby

Using ultrasound as a guide to the position of your baby, a needle is inserted into the amniotic sac and a sample of fluid is withdrawn.

Placenta

Uterus

Amniotic fluid

Cervix

Mucous plug

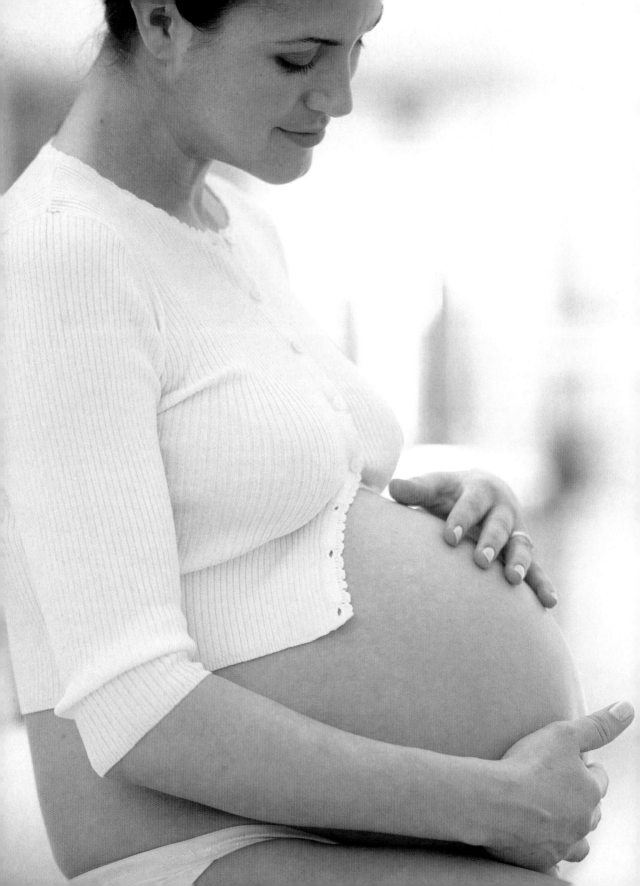

3RD TRIMESTER
what to expect

The very end of your pregnancy can be incredibly tiring. Your bump can get in the way of doing everyday things. It's time to relax as much as you can and save your energy for the birth.

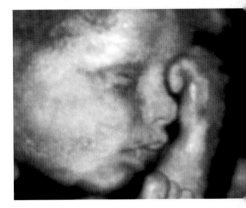

The perfectly formed features of a baby in the third trimester can be seen in this 3-dimensional ultrasound scan.

PHYSICAL CHANGES

Backaches, indigestion, swollen legs, difficulty sleeping, and needing to empty their bladders every 5 minutes, mean that most women count down to the birth of their babies in the last few weeks of pregnancy.

To cope with these physical discomforts, try to schedule your daily activities to accommodate for the slower moving last months, and allow for "nesting" time to prepare for your baby. If you haven't already done so, this is also a good time to plan with your partner the division of child care and housework after the birth.

Remaining a professional asset to your company to the very last day and communicating your maternity leave plans clearly will ensure a warm welcome back after maternity leave. However, if possible, lighten your workload progressively and take regular small breaks whenever you can to safeguard against exhaustion.

Physical activity and a good, nutritious diet through the end of your pregnancy keep you fit for birth, help speed up your recovery, and can prevent many of the discomforts of late pregnancy. During this trimester, medical care will include glucose testing to diagnose gestational diabetes and may include fetal heart monitoring to check your baby's health if your pregnancy is high risk.

YOUR BABY

During this trimester your baby will grow rapidly, up to 0.25kg (½lb) per week in the last month. Your baby's major organs will continue to mature, and more calcium builds up in your baby's bones, making them stronger.

While your baby is still breathing amniotic fluid, his or her lungs start to prepare for breathing air. Your baby's brain continues to grow and form more complex connections. Hearing progressively improves, and by the end of this trimester your baby starts to dream. By this point, your baby may have grown a full head of hair and is covered in a protective layer of thick, waxy material called vernix.

The third trimester is a **countdown to giving birth**. In the last few weeks, adapt what you do and **keep some reserves** for the birth.

your body

During the final 3 months of pregnancy, the major physical changes in your body are due to the increased size and weight of your baby. Many women find that this stage is incredibly uncomfortable, and the final weeks before delivery can seem like a lifetime. The baby presses on your bladder, and you may experience indigestion, breathlessness, and other common complaints.

GETTING THROUGH THE LAST FEW WEEKS

The end of pregnancy is appropriately called "misery of pregnancy" stage. Anyone who has been pregnant knows that the last few weeks of pregnancy would try the patience of a saint. Some of the discomforts are just that, a nuisance, but they are nothing to be worried about. Other changes in your body are more concerning and will need checking out.

Warning signs One of the things that often worsens in the last weeks is swelling in your feet and lower legs (see p105). Swelling is only worrisome if you have any new swelling in unexpected places, such as your hands and face, or if one of your legs suddenly swells more than the other. If any of these signs develop, call your care provider immediately. Rapid weight gain that occurs over the course of a few days is likely to be a sign of fluid retention and should also prompt you to call your midwife for advice.

APPETITE

Many women lose their appetite in the third trimester. There are several reasons for this. First and foremost is that, as your baby gets bigger, he or she pushes on your stomach, making it less easy to eat regular-sized meals. Second, acid reflux (indigestion, see p101) is at its highest level late in pregnancy, both because of the high levels of the hormone progesterone relaxing the opening between the stomach and the oesophagus, and because of greater pressure from the increasing size of the uterus. Eating less at this stage is not harmful to your baby.

You are likely to still be getting enough calories to maintain normal weight gain for your baby. At this point in your pregnancy, having regular snacks will help to maintain adequate intake of calories. You could also try spreading out your meals more during the day. In addition, make sure you are treating any symptoms of indigestion with antacids.

SLEEPING

Sleeping at night becomes very difficult in the late stages of pregnancy. It almost seems as if the last few weeks are a training period for the sleepless nights you will spend with your newborn. However, if at all possible, it helps to be well rested as you approach the marathon of labour. At this point in pregnancy, many

Lying on your side, with pillows under your legs, can help you sleep more easily at night.

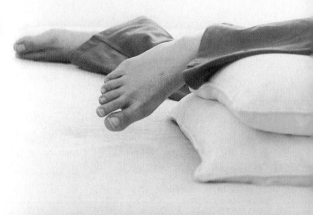

Dealing with a Fall

Given that movements can become clumsier in the third trimester, falls are quite common. In general, it is a good idea to be checked if you have a significant fall, even if there is no direct impact on your belly, because the placenta can be fragile in this trimester. The force of a fall can separate the placenta from the uterus. If you have fallen, your care provider will want to watch you for a few hours to make sure that you are not having contractions. You also may have a few blood tests, which can pick up any signs of bleeding in the placenta. If these blood tests are normal, you are not contracting, and your baby's heart rate monitoring is reassuring, it is unlikely that your fall has caused any problems for your baby.

women find that sleeping semi-reclined in a comfortable chair results in a better night's sleep.

Pile up the pillows Rounding up all the pillows in your house and creating a nest within your bed can also be an effective strategy to sleeping better, although your partner may feel squeezed out. Experiment as best you can, and make sure that acid reflux is treated so it doesn't keep you up at night. If less expensive measures fail, consider investing in a pregnancy body pillow — some women find these helpful. A final strategy is to have more short naps during the day if your routine allows.

PROBLEMS WITH WALKING

Many women find walking gets increasingly difficult late in the third trimester. Not only are you carrying a lot of extra weight, but your pelvis is changing. As you approach labour, the connections (ligaments) in your pelvis loosen and your pelvis becomes less stable. Some women notice shifting and pain at the connection at the front of the pelvis under the pubic hair (pelvic symphysis). This pain can be especially pronounced in women who have had several children.

As you negotiate this difficult time, walk slowly and get help as needed when sitting down and getting up. Don't force yourself to perform acrobatic feats to accomplish small tasks such as cutting your toenails — get help, professional or otherwise.

All your other joints also become more "loose" late in pregnancy, and this laxity — along with decreased agility at this stage of pregnancy — puts pregnant women at higher risk of joint injury. If you use common sense and extra care, you should be fine.

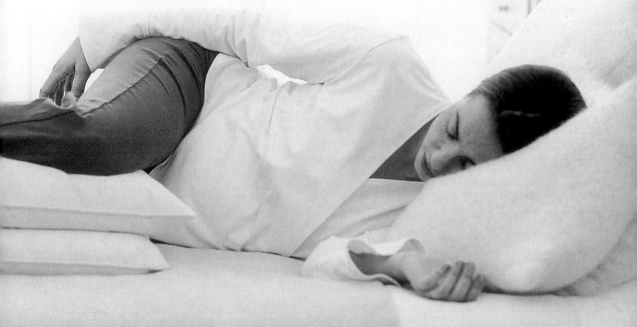

your emotions

The physical demands of the third trimester can exhaust your energy and deplete your emotional strength. As you prepare for the birth of your baby, you may have many conflicting emotions – excitement about holding your baby finally, fear of imminent labour, and worries about how you will cope. It's time to focus on this big event, to prepare for it both physically and mentally.

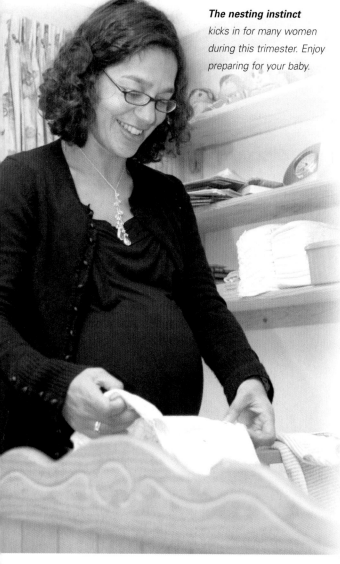

The nesting instinct kicks in for many women during this trimester. Enjoy preparing for your baby.

LOOKING AFTER YOUR NEEDS

As your baby grows quickly and your body changes in preparation for birth, you may encounter many physical discomforts, even if your pregnancy is healthy and trouble-free. Backaches, swollen legs and feet, stomach upsets, restless nights, clumsiness, and "baby brain" can turn even simple tasks into unpleasant chores.

At the same time as feeling physically drained, you may have a lot to do before the baby is born, and feel frustrated at your limited abilities. Try to lower your expectations of yourself to a realistic level. It is natural that you won't be at your most efficient or energetic just now. Don't beat yourself up.

Prioritizing It might help you feel more on top of your to-do list if you draw up a list of priorities. Focus on those things that absolutely need to be done before your baby is born, such as your medical check-ups and antenatal classes, packing your hospital bag, and making arrangements for other children during your stay in hospital. When you return from hospital you will need a handful of essential baby items such as a car seat, some nappies, a couple of sets of baby clothes, and a baby carrier so that you can be mobile from the start. Everything else can be bought and arranged after your baby has been born.

Focus also on the chores that give you pleasure. Shopping for clothes or toys for your baby can be a lot of fun, and getting the nursery ready for the new arrival can be very satisfying. If nesting brings you pleasure and some distraction from your aches and pains, indulge yourself, but at a leisurely pace.

Getting Ready to be a Single Parent

The last months of pregnancy can be especially emotionally taxing for you as a single parent. Attending antenatal classes and the usual drain of late pregnancy can highlight the fact that you are handling everything from medical decisions, to your baby's layette, to financial and career concerns all by yourself.

If you have not done so yet, it is important that you find a reliable support person for these last weeks of your pregnancy and for the birth of your baby. Take special care to cut your daily obligations to a minimum and to schedule your relaxation periods as a priority from now on.

Rest Your experience of this trimester — and possibly of the birth — will be greatly improved if you can manage to get as much rest and relaxation as possible. This means both mental and physical rest. Having a baby is hard work and your body may feel the strain of this work more quickly than the body of a younger woman, especially if you were out of shape before pregnancy. However, very few women have the luxury of being perfectly rested for the births of their babies, so if you don't have the time to put your feet up every day, don't let this alarm you because it causes no harm to the baby.

Buying clothes that fit and look nice Towards the end of pregnancy it can feel unreasonable to spend money on new maternity clothes. However, with the physical discomforts of late pregnancy and the dwindling grace in movement, well-fitting, comfortable clothes can help you maintain a positive attitude. To get more value for your money, look for styles that allow you to breastfeed easily, if this is your intention.

PREPARING FOR LABOUR

Focusing on the birth is natural at this time. Fear and anxiety about the big transition you are about to experience are also natural, even if this is not your first baby. You will feel more in control and centred if you are emotionally and mentally prepared for labour. Read as much as you can about the birth process so you are familiar with the different stages of labour (see p124–125) and have an idea of what to expect. Also, practise birthing positions that look and feel comfortable to you, and breathing exercises to help you cope with contractions.

Make sure your birth partners know your wishes regarding the birth. Tell them which medical interventions you are happy with and which ones you hope to avoid, where and how you hope to give birth, and suggest ways in which your birth partners can help you feel as comfortable as possible at the time. This will help you feel confident that you will receive the support you need during labour.

Trust your body Be reassured by the fact that you are not the first woman in the world to give birth. Billions of other women through the ages have done what you are about to do, and with a lot less medical expertise and assistance at hand than you have.

The female body has evolved to be capable of childbirth, and your natural instincts may well guide you when your brain is at a loss in the situation. You are biologically ready for labour, even if you may not feel as if you are. Try to trust your body and have confidence in its innate birthing skills.

fear and **excitement** mingle as you approach **labour** and finally **meeting your baby**

Look after yourself Your emotions at this time are likely to be complex and somewhat volatile, so make time to pamper yourself and think about what you need most now — you may want some time alone reading books or reflecting on your baby, or you may want to spend more time with friends.

your relationships

Unless you already have a child, the last 3 months of your pregnancy are also your last 3 months as a twosome, so enjoy your present situation to the full before a new chapter of your life begins. These are also months of intense preparation for the arrival of your baby. You will take antenatal classes, shop for baby items, and make plans for the birth itself.

After the birth of your baby, you and your partner will always have to consider the needs of another person in your family. The dynamics of your daily lives will change dramatically, especially in the first few months when your baby demands your full attention and you adjust to caring for him or her.

Therefore, you may want to schedule special times just for you and your partner into these last weeks of pregnancy. Do things you enjoy doing together that will be limited while your baby is very young. Go out to dinner, visit museums, go away for a romantic weekend, go and see lots of movies, and spend plenty of time talking (after all, a good deal of your conversation will soon be about the baby). Appreciate how the beginning of your partnership has changed your lives in a big way, and consider how the arrival of your baby is about to change your lives again.

PREPARING FOR LABOUR TOGETHER

The thought of the birth may elicit both excitement and fear in you. The thrill of finally holding your child stands in stark contrast to the uncertainty about the onset, length, and painfulness of your labour.

Men often worry about their ability to be truly helpful during labour and how they may react when they see their baby being born. Older parents might harbour fears of having an unhealthy baby. If this is your first birth experience, it is particularly important that you and your partner are able to share your hopes and fears openly with one another. Talk about how you are feeling about the birth, and listen to your partner's perspective. You don't need to

handle this alone, and your partner need not live with his fears alone. You can manage the birth of your baby together.

Participating in antenatal classes with your partner can help to make the impending birth and subsequent care of your baby more of a reality for you both, and help you plan for giving birth and parenting. Consider now that your expectations of how events will proceed in the hours and days after the birth may not match your partner's. For example, you may want him to stay

working with your partner **towards a good labour** will help you feel supported

with you while he plans to return to work and share the news with his colleagues. Exchanging these ideas and clarifying the needs both of you have now will enable you to support one another most effectively at this significant turning point in your lives.

Your partner's role As more of your strength is required to maintain your baby's growth, it's important that your partner takes on some preparations for your baby's arrival. For some men, this is the start of putting time and effort into the baby, and it can be a hard step.

It's important that your partner commits to caring for your new baby. Parenting is hard work, demanding much of your time and energy. If you are both to continue working, it is vital that your partner invests time and effort in parenting, giving you equal time and energy to invest in your career. Prepare yourself to help him adjust to the new demands placed on him. Taking part in the last preparations before birth may be a natural start for his involvement.

Once the baby is born, some men don't take on as much babycare as they had intended to once the reality of the situation dawns on them. Give your partner clear, practical guidelines as to what will be expected of him. Agree now on tasks to designate to him, and write down your agreement so that you both have a reminder of it once the baby is born. Then hold him to it! No one enjoys housework, so both of you will probably have some complaints and small struggles. However, a clear and fair division of tasks should keep renegotiation to a minimum.

The timing of birth is usually unpredictable. Babies can arrive two weeks earlier or later and be considered on time. If you want your partner to be at the birth, communicate clearly that his presence and assistance is needed as early in the process as possible. For many women, reassurance from their partners that they will be there as soon as needed calms their fears of labour considerably. Suggest that he arrange in advance to allow for a sudden departure from work.

INVOLVING YOUR CHILDREN

The last months of your pregnancy are the perfect time to prepare older siblings for the arrival of your baby. Much sibling rivalry can be prevented by assigning older siblings the role of insightful caretaker of their new baby sister or brother (this information must be presented more than once to younger children) and by allowing them to make some of the decisions about baby clothes, blankets, and toys. You might like to plan a gift for your child, to present on the day of the birth to thank him or her for being such a good big brother or sister.

Reassuring your child Bear in mind that young children often regress right before birth in an attempt to get your attention. In the third trimester,

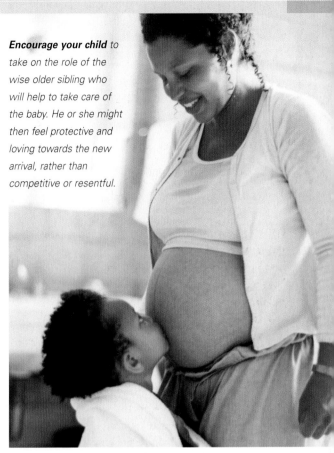

Encourage your child to take on the role of the wise older sibling who will help to take care of the baby. He or she might then feel protective and loving towards the new arrival, rather than competitive or resentful.

you'll find it hard to pick up your toddler, and he or she will need lots of cuddles to make up for this. Give your child plenty of reassurance, and don't stress potty training, for example, too hard at this time.

Children need to know how they will be taken care of when you birth your baby. They need to understand who will take them to or pick them up from school, prepare meals in your absence, and whether they will be able to see you and the new baby at the hospital or birth centre. They will also need to know when you will return home after the new baby has been born. You may want to ask older children which arrangements they would prefer and allow them to take an active part in making these plans a reality.

If your child is to be present at the birth, tell him or her about the sights and sounds of giving birth. Let him or her know that you will be in pain, but that this is perfectly natural so there is no cause for alarm.

your career

Depending on your general health and the level of stress in your life, you may experience the last trimester of your pregnancy as an intensely taxing time or as the welcome conclusion of an exciting process. Your physical and emotional wellbeing will dictate how you tackle the last months at work, but whatever the case, try to control your workload and plan ahead for your maternity leave.

Whether you are feeling fit and well or are struggling to keep all the threads of your life going, try to keep two objectives in mind during your last months at work. First, make sure that you work and leave well so that your colleagues and your boss are happy to see you when you return. Second, reduce your workload and stress level so that you have time and emotional space to prepare for your baby's arrival.

MAINTAIN CONTROL

During your last months at work, aim to look and act professional. Although you may find the physical strain of the final weeks of your pregnancy challenging – and your mind may be much more on the impending birth of your baby than work – the impression you make at work is important for your plans to return after the birth. Your composure in the last weeks before maternity leave can translate into favourable options later, such as more flexible working patterns, that only a trusted employee may enjoy.

Sometimes, colleagues and employers may discount your ability to get things done when you are looking so heavily pregnant. Important projects may be given to non-pregnant colleagues and you may miss out on chances to advance your career. If you are reasonably

start **handing over** some of your responsibilities before you leave

confident that you can contribute to or even manage a project and if it would have fallen into your area of responsibilities, insist that it be given to you. If your pregnancy is proceeding without significant problems, there is no reason for you to be treated any less favourably than before you became pregnant.

PLAN YOUR DEPARTURE

If you can choose to take on projects you know you can complete before your maternity leave begins, opt for these. If you are part of a team, negotiate for aspects of the whole effort that you can finish in your time left at work. Completing self-contained assignments will increase the likelihood that you receive due credit for your contributions, even while you are on leave.

Sick Leave in Pregnancy

If you are unable to work because of pregnancy-related illness, your employer should still pay you in the same way as if you were not pregnant. However, if you need to stop work for a medical reason within 4 weeks of your due date, you are obliged to start your maternity leave. (You can actually start maternity leave up to 11 weeks before your due date.) Your employer should record pregnancy-related sickness separately from normal sick leave as it would be considered discriminatory to take into account pregnancy-related absences when calculating length of sickness absence, for example in your performance appraisal or selection for redundancy.

Control your workload Creating balance between your career life and the demands of your pregnancy is essential in the weeks leading up to the birth of your baby. Having a baby is probably the most challenging thing you will ever do and you need to maintain good physical and emotional reserves for it. Your goals of maintaining a professional demeanour and delivering quality work up to your last day at work are best achieved by controlling your workload.

Communicate your plans for maternity leave Most people don't like living with uncertainty. Your boss and your colleagues will appreciate knowing the details of your maternity leave, especially if they are going to be directly affected by an increased workload due to your absence. Openly communicating the aspects of your maternity leave that pertain to those who work with you gives them the opportunity to rearrange their plans for the coming months. It also provides a timeframe for the orderly transfer of your responsibilities to others.

Show your appreciation Pregnancy is such an all-encompassing event that it can be easy to lose track of how it affects those around us. The reality in most companies is that your colleagues will be asked to pick up the work you leave behind during your absence.

Co-workers usually appreciate that you acknowledge their contribution on your behalf. How you show your gratitude is an individual matter. A word of thanks, or helping someone become familiar with one of your tasks, can make a big difference.

STARTING MATERNITY LEAVE

Depending on your position at work, you may be able to select someone to continue your projects while you are on leave. There may be one person who is most familiar with your responsibilities and can become the point of contact for any questions or concerns that would usually be directed to you. Make sure that he or she is well informed and has clear instructions for the successful completion of any task you have begun.

Give your home contact information to one person only. Even if you feel you want to be helpful while you are at work, when you are home with your new baby you will probably welcome privacy and rest. Phone calls from your place of work are likely to be disruptive and unwelcome. Inform your co-workers who will have your contact information and make sure that everyone understands that you are to be contacted by this person only.

Continuing responsibilities Women in prominent positions in their company often need to continue performing at their best right up until they leave.

exercise programme

Towards the end of pregnancy, you'll feel bulky and very tired, and once your baby drops into his or her birth position, you may have trouble just walking, let alone exercising! But persevere if you can – there are many physical benefits for women who continue to exercise regularly in the third trimester.

Your body is doing a lot of extra work right now. By the end of pregnancy, your heart pumps one and a half times as much blood and beats 15 times more per minute than before pregnancy. Some conditions of late pregnancy, and carrying multiple babies, are reason to stop moderate activity in the third trimester. Therefore, always clear continued exercise with your healthcare provider.

Benefits of Exercise

There are many ways in which exercise can improve your well-being in the third trimester.

- **Swollen legs and ankles**
  Swelling is usually due to poor circulation and sluggish metabolism processes. Exercise, especially swimming, can provide relief.

- **Constipation** Exercise increases your metabolic rate, and speeds up nutrient and waste processing.

- **Labour and recovery after birth**
  Women who exercise regularly often have shorter, easier labours with fewer complications, and faster recovery periods after birth.

RECOMMENDED EXERCISES

The weight of your baby and the restriction of your movement may limit the types of exercise you can do now. Swimming and water activities are ideal because they support your weight and encourage blood flow back to your heart.

EXERCISING SAFELY

A few safety measures will allow you to take care of yourself and your baby during exercise.

Choosing safe activities Most low-impact movements are safe during this trimester. Your baby's weight now puts much strain on your bones and muscles, including the lower back and pelvic muscles, which are relaxing in preparation for labour. The enzymes that loosen your pelvis loosen other joints, too, so you are at higher risk of joint injury. Avoid bouncy exercise such as jogging or high-impact aerobics. Replace these with an alternative – speed walking can replace jogging, for instance.

Reduce intensity Your physical activity should make you feel invigorated and refreshed. If that is not the case, you are over-exerting yourself, so find a less taxing alternative. Cut short or skip your workout if you are tired.

Avoid high-risk sports Injuries to your belly can be serious, so avoid activities involving a risk of falling, contact sports, extreme sports, and ball games. These require balance and coordination. Neither can be relied on as your belly takes its final shape and weight. By the end of pregnancy, your body has an additional burden of up to 18kg (40lb), which is largely concentrated at the front of your body. Allow for your shifting centre of gravity.

Swimming is ideal for late pregnancy. Allowing the water to support your weight can be a pleasant and rejuvenating relief.

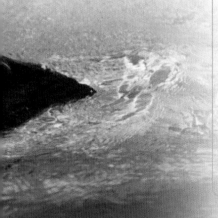

IDEAL EXERCISES FOR THE 3RD TRIMESTER

Exercise	Benefits and suggestions	Frequency and duration
Swimming	Swim with long, measured strokes or just try floating on your back. To be ready for this relaxing activity, look for a swimsuit during the summer months; it may be difficult to find one later on.	Daily if possible, or four to five times a week. Do what is comfortable, but 20–30 minutes is ideal.
Water aerobics	A water aerobics class offers a more structured setting for regular physical activity at a time when you may not be terribly motivated to exercise. It's also a great way of getting a gentle aerobic workout.	Three or four times a week if you feel able to. If classes are longer than 30 to 45 minutes stop before you become too tired.
Reclined cycle workouts	As your belly undergoes its final growth spurt, a reclining bike may be more comfortable than an upright one. If you start to feel dizzy at all, stop.	Several times a week if you feel able to. If this is the only exercise you do, then aim for 20–30 minute sessions.
Tai-chi	The slow, flowing moves of tai-chi may be ideal for you during the last trimester. These moves will help you relax and preserve your energy for the birth of your baby.	Daily sessions of 10–30 minutes are ideal. Two or three times a week will offer significant benefits.
Kegel exercises	Doing Kegel exercises to work your pelvic floor muscles enables them to stretch fully during delivery and contract completely afterwards. To find which muscles to contract, try stopping the flow of urine while you urinate. Once you know how, you can perform these muscle tightenings anywhere.	For best results, exercise several times throughout the day. It's good to do these while you are waiting at a red traffic light, for example. Aim for 5 sets of 10 repetitions, as these muscles get tired, too.

food plan

As your baby's nutritional needs increase during this final growth spurt, you are more at risk of developing nutritional deficiencies. Your body is designed to make sure that your baby's needs are met before your own. A balanced diet providing the extra calories needed each day throughout pregnancy can protect you while making sure your baby gets all he or she needs.

During the last trimester, the nutritional needs of your baby can be met best with a balanced diet supplemented with antenatal vitamins. In particular, make sure you're getting enough calcium and B vitamins – along with other minerals and vitamins that are important for both you and your baby (see p48 and p72).

Your life may seem busier than ever in these weeks, and preparing meals may seem time-consuming. But make sure that you don't skip mealtimes, so that you maintain your energy levels. Focus on getting servings from all food groups (dairy products, vegetables, meat and fish, fruits, grains and cereals.) If you feel uncomfortable, especially if you have heartburn and bloating, reduce meal sizes, and have regular snacks. Choose foods that are high in nutritional value rather than calories. The best way to make sure you don't put on too much weight while you are pregnant is with a sensible eating plan and by keeping as active as possible. If you think you are putting on too much weight, don't be tempted to restrict your intake significantly without the supervision of your healthcare provider. You may want to ask your care provider about visiting a trained nutritionist.

VITAMINS AND MINERALS

A well-balanced diet will provide you with all the vitamins and minerals you need to keep you healthy and the baby growing well. During the third trimester, your baby will reach his or her birth weight and will need higher amounts of B vitamin complex and calcium. Both are essential for the development of your baby's blood supply and skeleton. These key nutritional components can make a difference to your health, too.

B vitamin complex Vitamins B_1 (thiamin), B_2 (riboflavin), B_3 (niacin), B_6, B_{12}, pantothenic acid, and folic acid (see p22) are all part of the B vitamin complex. These vitamins occur together in foods and enhance your body's nerve function and help the release of energy from foods. Vitamins B_6 and B_{12} are of special significance because they aid in the formation of red blood cells.

Both you and your baby also need these two vitamins to extract nutrients from any of the foods you eat and for nervous system development and health. To cover your requirements for B vitamins, eat wholegrain foods. Enriched cereals and rice are other good sources. Note that meat, fish,

Fruit salad provides lots of vitamins and makes a nutritious snack. A topping of yogurt adds calcium.

poultry, and dairy products are the only sources of vitamin B_{12}, so vegans must take supplements to get adequate B_{12}.

Calcium This mineral is needed at all stages of pregnancy, but in the last few weeks it is needed in greater amounts to help your baby's teeth and bones develop. Calcium is also important for your own health, reducing bone loss during pregnancy and therefore protecting you from developing

The RDA for calcium during pregnancy is 1,200–1,500mg. Antenatal vitamins contain only 40–200mg of calcium, and calcium supplements contain less than one-third of the RDA. If you do choose to take a supplement, bear in mind that you will still need to consume calcium-rich foods.

ESSENTIAL FLUIDS
Fluids help deliver nutrients to your baby, flush away waste products, and build your baby's blood supply and

> ## nutrients in your diet interact with one another to grow your baby and keep you both healthy

serious osteoporosis (bone loss) in later life. If you don't have enough calcium in your diet while you are pregnant there is a chance that you may lose calcium from your bones to provide enough for your baby. You can get enough calcium by eating at least three servings of dairy products daily. However, whole grains, green leafy vegetables, eggs, and nuts are also good sources (see right.)

Supplements The recommended daily allowance (RDA) for B vitamins during pregnancy are: B_1, 1.5mg; B_2, 1.6mg; B_3, 17mg; B_6, 2.2mg; folic acid, 400 mcg; B_{12}, 2.2mcg. In general, antenatal vitamins contain adequate amounts of these B vitamins.

body cells. These fluids are best supplied by water. Drink enough to make sure that your urine is a pale straw colour. Bright yellow or dark urine is a sign you are not getting enough water.

USING DIET TO COPE WITH LATE PREGNANCY PROBLEMS
Diet can be a useful tool in helping control some of the discomforts of late pregnancy (see p100–107). For example, if you have constipation and haemorrhoids, eat foods rich in fibre, such as bran breakfast cereals or dried prunes. Keep your meal schedule predictable, and drink fluids throughout the day.

If you have gestational diabetes, follow the dietary guidelines given by your doctor or nutritionist.

Sources of B_6 and B_{12}

Vitamins B_6 and B_{12} are particularly important in aiding the formation of red blood cells. The following foods are good sources of vitamin B_6:

- beef and pork
- fish and poultry
- bread and brown rice
- baked potato (with skin)
- egg yolks
- bananas
- prune juice and carrot juice
- nuts and peanut butter
- chickpeas.

Vitamin B_{12} rich foods include the following:

- pork, lamb, and beef
- eggs and dairy products
- white fish and salmon
- fortified cereals.

Sources of Calcium

It's important to have adequate calcium to build your baby's teeth and skeleton and maintain your own bone structure. These foods are good sources:

- dairy products
- sardines and salmon
- soya beans and tofu
- almonds, hazel nuts, and brazil nuts
- sesame seeds.

Calcium is also present in smaller amounts in leafy green vegetables, oranges, and dried figs.

antenatal care

In the last 3 months of pregnancy you can expect to be seen by your doctor or midwife with increasing frequency. Check-ups at this critical stage of pregnancy are very important because it is a time when problems can develop. Frequent visits ensure that both you and your baby are doing well, and that any problems that do develop are quickly picked up.

Generally, you should expect to be seen every 2–3 weeks in the early third trimester. Between 36 weeks and the time you deliver, visits will increase depending on how you are. Problems such as preeclampsia (see p113) or problems with your placenta that can cause your baby's growth to slow down, are most likely to become apparent in this trimester. You are likely to have various tests, either as part of your routine visits or separately.

ROUTINE CHECK-UPS
Your blood pressure, weight, and urine will be tested at each visit. High blood pressure can develop in pregnancy and, in some cases, can represent the early stages of preeclampsia. Your doctor tests your urine for signs of protein (none or trace is okay) and glucose. High protein levels can be a sign of preeclampsia. Excess glucose can mean you are getting gestational diabetes (see p110).

Weight Your doctor or midwife may monitor your weight gain. This is done to check you aren't putting on too much weight, which could cause complications late in your pregnancy. (However, your weight doesn't reflect your baby's growth.)

Blood tests Only a few blood tests are performed in this trimester and not all of them are done routinely. If you are thought to

THIRD TRIMESTER TESTS

Type of test	When it is done	What results show
Blood test	Approximately 28 weeks	Blood sample is taken and tested for whether you are anaemic; it is also tested for antibodies, especially if you are Rhesus negative. (The sample may be taken at the same time as that taken for the glucose tolerance test.)
Urine test	At each visit	Sample tested for presence of protein in urine, which may be a sign of preeclampsia (see p113) and glucose, which may indicate diabetes (see p110).
Glucose tolerance test	28 weeks (if necessary)	Blood sample is taken just before, then 1 and 2 hours after drinking a super-sweet drink. Results indicate whether you have gestational diabetes (see p110).
Fetal heart monitoring	Usually starting at 32 weeks, if needed	Two monitors placed on abdomen check uterine contractions and baby's heart rate. (Only done in women with conditions that may affect placental blood flow or who are high risk for other reasons.)

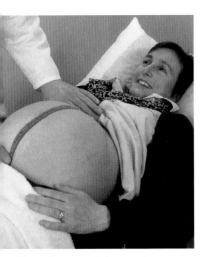

Measuring your abdomen gives your doctor an easy way of checking your baby is growing properly.

be at risk of gestational diabetes, you will have a glucose tolerence test. Gestational diabetes is more common in women over 35.

This test involves drinking a very sweet drink containing sugar. A blood sample is drawn 1 and 2 hours afterwards and tested for the glucose level. A result of less than 7.8g/l is considered normal. A positive test identifies women who have glucose intolerance. If you have a positive test, you will need to check your sugar levels in daily life until the baby is born.

As well as your glucose test, a blood sample may be checked to make sure that you are recovering from second trimester anaemia. If not, your care provider may want you to take extra iron tablets.

Finally, in most cases, your care provider may also check your blood for antibodies that can affect your baby's blood count; this test is especially important for women who are Rhesus negative.

If you are Rhesus negative you should also receive an injection of anti-D at around 28 weeks and 34 weeks gestation to protect you from developing harmful antibodies.

CHECKING YOUR BABY'S GROWTH

Your baby's growth is monitored by measuring your uterus at each visit; this test is called the fundal height. In general, your fundal height in centimetres should equal the number of weeks pregnant you are (after 20 weeks). If there are any concerns your doctor may order an extra ultrasound.

MONITORING YOUR BABY

While the tests described above are important for a healthy pregnancy, other tests are done specifically to monitor your baby's well-being inside your uterus.

Kick charts These are a way for you to check that your baby is moving well. If you feel your baby move all the time you don't need to perform kick charts. But, because women often don't notice whether their baby is moving when they are busy, kick charts are a great way to reassure yourself if you are uncertain. Each day you should count your baby's movements to 10 and note the time at which 10 movements were achieved. This should be about the same each day. If you

haven't felt movement by your usual time, you should call the hospital for advice.

Fetal heart monitoring Two tests, fetal heart monitoring and biophysical profile (BPP), check to make sure that your baby is getting enough nutrients and oxygen through your placenta.

If you have a medical condition that can affect the blood flow in your placenta, such as high blood pressure, diabetes, or systemic lupus (see p18) your doctor will probably order one of these tests once or twice a week after about 32 weeks of pregnancy.

With fetal heart monitoring (also known as a CTG recording), two monitors are placed on your abdomen. One checks for uterine contractions, the other listens to your baby's heart rate. The test is "reassuring" if your baby's heart rate speeds up twice in a 20–30 minute test, and there are no big dips. If your baby has a nonreactive CTG (where the heart rate doesn't speed up) it may mean that your baby is just asleep. Your doctor will then listen to your baby's heart for a bit longer or order a biophysical profile (BPP). A BPP is an ultrasound test combined with heart rate monitoring that checks four criteria: amniotic fluid volume, fetal movement, fetal tone and breathing movements. A reassuring result with BPP or fetal heart monitoring means that your baby is at low risk of a problem over the next week.

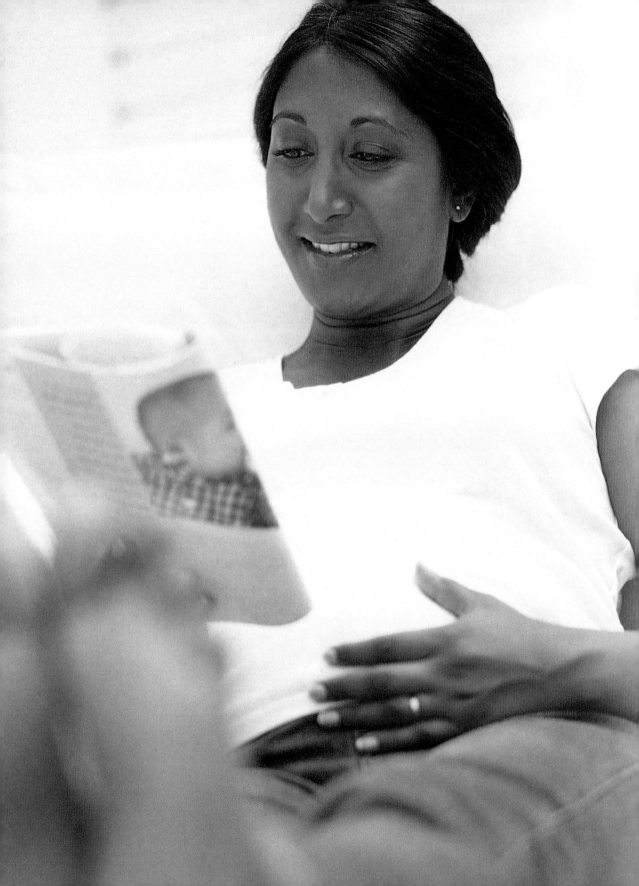

COMMON COMPLAINTS

Pregnancy brings with it a raft of physical changes, most of which are not particularly pleasant. While causing some women considerable misery, most are not signs of a serious problem.

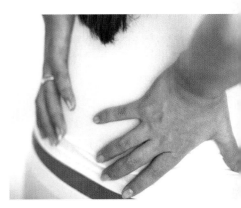

Common pregnancy complaints are especially trying for women over 35. Older women may interpret some of the discomforts of pregnancy as more severe because of their age. Most of the time this is not the case. Younger women have all of the same complaints and problems that you will experience, although in some instances your age may make the symptoms worse or make it more likely that you will experience a particular symptom.

GENERAL PHYSICAL HEALTH

Pregnancy may exacerbate some of the general physical problems that tend to become more common as we age. For example, back pain is common in pregnancy but also increases as we age. Women need to take especially good care of their backs during pregnancy; back-strengthening exercises, careful lifting technique, and

Swollen legs and ankles are especially common in the later stages of pregnancy. Resting with your feet raised helps to reduce this swelling.

workplace modifications are especially important.

Stress incontinence, which is the involuntary loss of urine with coughing or laughing, is more common as we age and can first appear during pregnancy. For this reason, doing pelvic floor exercises can be especially important in older mothers.

As we age, our skin loses its elasticity and may be more sensitive to some of the changes caused by pregnancy, possibly including such things as stretch marks. If you have been pregnant before, you may notice more pelvic pain in this pregnancy because of loosening and shifting of your pelvic ligaments.

TREATING PROBLEMS

Your care provider can provide useful tips for dealing with most minor complaints of pregnancy. Often, simple measures are helpful – such as raising your legs if your legs and ankles are swollen. Always check with your doctor before taking any medication, even over-the-counter products.

Back pain is a common problem, affecting 50 per cent of women during pregnancy. It is more likely in older women and those in their second or subsequent pregnancies.

Common **pregnancy complaints** are particularly trying for **women over 35**, but most can be **easily alleviated**.

minor pregnancy complaints

Most women experience some discomforts during pregnancy, and often these are worse in the later stages. There is nearly always something you can do or take to ease these problems. However, it is important to remember that certain commonly used over-the-counter medications should not be used in pregnancy. Always ask your doctor before taking over-the-counter remedies.

HEADACHES

Some women have headaches that are often aggravated by hormonal changes with their menstrual cycles. These women may notice an increase in headaches during pregnancy, but this is uncommon.

The first line of treatment for a headache in pregnancy should be a product that contains pure paracetamol. Products that contain aspirin or nonsteroidal anti-inflammatory agents (NSAIDs) such as ibuprofen should be avoided because of the risks of affecting the baby. If you suffer migraines, you may need prescription medication. However, don't take serotonin receptor agonists such as sumatriptan because these can reduce blood flow to the placenta. If necessary, severe migraine pain can be treated safely with opioid analgesics such as codeine. Beta-blocking agents can be continued to be used to prevent migraines if necessary.

In general, migraines tend to improve during pregnancy and most women have complete remission from headaches or a significant decrease in symptoms. If you have a severe headache in the last trimester of pregnancy and you don't normally suffer from severe headaches, you should call the hospital straight away, especially if you also have visual changes such as flashes of light or blurred vision. This could be a sign of preeclampsia (see p113).

▶ **WHAT'S SAFE TO USE** Paracetamol; some beta-blocker drugs; opioid analgesics

▶ **WHAT TO AVOID** Aspirin; ibuprofen and other NSAIDs.

NASAL STUFFINESS

Many women notice increased nasal congestion when they are pregnant. This stuffiness is due to the increase in blood flow to the mucous membranes in the nose. The hormone oestrogen causes an increase in mucous secretion during pregnancy. Increased blood flow to the fragile blood vessels in your nose also makes nose bleeds very common. While the increased congestion is annoying, it is quite normal and will not interfere with the amount of oxygen that your baby receives. Avoid using nasal sprays (except pure saline) because they tend to cause even more nasal stuffiness if you do not use them constantly. If you find it hard to sleep, you may get some relief by using a humidifier at night.

▶ **WHAT'S SAFE TO USE** Diphenhydramine; phenylephedrine

▶ **WHAT TO AVOID** Nasal sprays

DIZZINESS

During pregnancy, most of your blood vessels dilate (widen) to allow unrestricted blood flow to the uterus and your baby. This produces a small drop in blood pressure and may increase the chances that you feel dizzy. Pregnant women are especially sensitive to changes in position, and you are most likely to feel dizzy when you stand up too quickly. Try to avoid rapid changes in position, and sit back down if you feel dizzy. Dizziness on its own is not a sign of a health problem. As your pregnancy progresses, you may also notice you feel dizzy when you lie on your back. This is because the uterus presses down and cuts off blood returning from your lower body to your heart. Lying on your side should alleviate this dizziness. If your dizziness comes on after heart palpitations, or if it is not relieved by lying on your side, consult your doctor.

BLEEDING GUMS

Most women notice that during pregnancy their gums are much more likely to bleed after being brushed. This is normal and results from the increase in blood flow to the gums in pregnancy. However, it's important you look after your teeth properly. Gum disease, for example, may be associated with problems such as preterm labour. If you have not seen your dentist recently, it is safe to have your teeth cleaned or have a filling, but try to avoid dental X-rays unless necessary.

PALPITATIONS

Heart palpitations, recognizable by the feeling that your heart has missed a beat or "flip flops" inside your chest, seem to be more common and more noticeable during pregnancy. Generally, palpitations are not serious if they happen only occasionally and you don't have other symptoms such as dizziness. If you do have other symptoms, discuss them with your doctor straight away.

BREAST TENDERNESS AND ENLARGEMENT

Over the course of pregnancy, you can expect that each breast will "gain" up to 0.5kg (1lb) in weight. During pregnancy your breasts may be quite tender, especially in the first trimester. While all of these changes are normal, they mean that you should wear a good bra for support. Early in pregnancy you can wear a sports bra (even to bed). In the second trimester, it is a good idea to invest in a couple of pregnancy or nursing bras at around the same time as you move into maternity clothes. Remember to continue your monthly breast examinations during this period, and bring any noticeable lumps to the attention of your doctor.

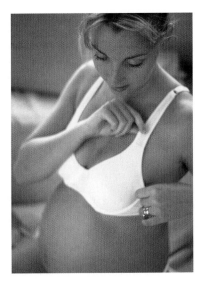

Support bras are a great help in reducing breast tenderness, even in early pregnancy, and can be worn to bed, too.

BREATHLESSNESS

The hormone progesterone affects how you breathe while you are pregnant, making your breaths deeper and more rapid than normal. A common side-effect of these changes is a feeling of breathlessness. Shortness of breath increases with exertion, such as walking up a flight of stairs. This feeling is normal, and does not mean that you are out of shape, too old to have a baby, or that you have a problem with your heart or lungs. As your baby gets bigger, you are likely to notice that you become more and more breathless, and may get worse when you try to lie flat. Some women find that they need to sleep partially sitting up towards the end of pregnancy.

INDIGESTION

Progesterone, the hormone of pregnancy, relaxes the smooth muscle of the uterus allowing your pregnancy to grow. At the same time, other smooth muscle is relaxed. One of the unpleasant side-effects is the relaxation of the opening between your stomach and your oesophagus (the tube between your mouth and stomach). Combine this with slowly increasing pressure on your stomach from your growing uterus and you have the potential for raging indigestion. Contrary to common belief, what you eat has only a small effect, although eating a large meal may make your symptoms worse. The main factors that worsen indigestion are the acidity of your stomach contents and your position (for example, lying down or standing).

Antacids are good for reducing the acid content of your stomach. Most over-the-counter antacids are safe in pregnancy and products that contain calcium are especially good. However, many women need stronger antacids or histamine receptor antagonists (H$_2$ blockers), which you can get from chemists or on prescription. You can also help ease indigestion by not lying down or bending over immediately after a meal.

▶ **WHAT'S SAFE TO USE** Histamine receptor antagonists (H$_2$ blockers); antacids containing calcium carbonate or magnesium carbonate

ABDOMINAL PAIN

Almost all pregnant women will have some abdominal pains during their pregnancy. The trick is knowing if the pain is a sign of something more serious. Early in pregnancy, many women feel uterine cramping, pelvic pressure, and generalized mild abdominal discomfort. This results from a combination of your uterus reacting to the pregnancy and the effects of the rising levels of the hormone progesterone on your intestines. As you enter the second trimester, nonspecific abdominal pains are common. Most are from

---

Warning Signs

In the first trimester of pregnancy, abdominal pain accompanied by any of the following should prompt you to see your doctor:

- vaginal bleeding that is more than spotting
- fever greater than 39°C (100.4°F)
- history of ectopic pregnancy or you currently have an IUD in place
- burning when you pass urine.

In the second trimester, call your doctor if abdominal pain occurs with:

- any vaginal bleeding, even spotting
- a noticeable increase in vaginal discharge, especially a lot of watery or mucous discharge
- a fever higher than 39°C (100.4°F)
- vaginal pressure.

---

gassiness and bloating. Pains along the sides of your uterus, caused by stretching of the uterine supports (round ligament pain), are also common. As you progress in your third trimester, it is common to have an increase in uterine activity, or Braxton-Hicks contractions. These contractions are felt as a tightening sensation across your uterus and should not be particularly painful. If you have painful contractions across the front of your uterus, or you have lower back pain that comes and goes, call your care provider – especially if you are less than 34 weeks gestation.

▶ **WHAT'S SAFE TO USE** Paracetamol

GAS PAINS AND BLOATING

The action of progesterone slows down the workings of your intestines and can lead to bloating. Most of the gas comes from the action of bacteria on carbohydrates in your diet; the slower your intestines move food through, the more time bacteria have to digest the food and the more gas is produced. If you are having problems with gas, start by avoiding foods that are more likely to produce gas, such as beans, cauliflower, broccoli, and cabbage.

Avoid carbonated beverages that may increase the amount of gas in your intestines, but increase the amount of water you drink. Taking a walk after meals may help to stimulate your digestive tract naturally.

▶ **WHAT'S SAFE TO USE** Over-the-counter medications containing simethicone are thought to be safe

THRUSH INFECTIONS

Although pregnancy is not associated with an increase in vaginal thrush infection, many women who suffer from recurrent thrush infections are concerned about using anti-fungal medications during pregnancy. Over-the-counter thrush creams and pessaries are safe during pregnancy. If your doctor has asked you not to put anything in

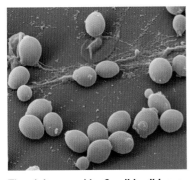

Thrush is caused by Candida albicans, *a fungal yeast that occurs normally in moist areas of the body.*

your vagina because you have a placenta praevia, you can avoid using the applicator and place the cream on the vulval lips and the lower part of your vagina. If your thrush infection does not get better, your doctor may want to confirm the infection and treat it with other drugs.

▶ **WHAT'S SAFE TO USE** Over-the-counter yeast creams such as clotrimazole

URINARY INCONTINENCE

Up to half of women have a problem with involuntary loss of urine during pregnancy. Certainly, in the first trimester you will notice you have the urge to urinate often. This urgency decreases by the second trimester, but you will still have to empty your bladder more often than before you were pregnant. Incontinence is most common in the third trimester, especially if you have had problems with urine loss in the

past or you have been pregnant before. Usually the amount of urine lost is small and wearing a pad should be enough to catch any accidents. Women who have incontinence while pregnant are more likely to have problems later.

If you suddenly start "leaking" and have been fine before, make sure your doctor or midwife rules out a possible urinary tract infection, which may be causing the incontinence.

If your symptoms don't resolve by 3 months after delivery, consider seeing a specialist. In some cases of overactive bladder, medication to relax your bladder spasms can reduce accidents. In other cases, surgical or nonsurgical treatment, such as physiotherapy, is needed.

CONSTIPATION AND HAEMORRHOIDS

The slowing action of progesterone on your large intestine increases water absorption, leaving you with harder stools. Pressure from your uterus also slows blood flow from the blood vessels around the rectum and anus, increasing haemorrhoids. This is not a good combination. The best way to combat these problems is to decrease constipation because straining can make haemorrhoids worse. The first step is to soften your stools by increasing water intake and taking

bulking agents. If this gentle method does not work, you can add stool softeners, reserving laxatives for serious cases of constipation. If haemorrhoids develop despite maintaining normal stool consistency, try to clean carefully after each bowel movement with a pad soaked in witch hazel. Haemorrhoid creams may also help to reduce swelling and are safe in pregnancy.

▶ **WHAT'S SAFE TO USE** Fibre or other bulking agents; stool softeners; laxatives; creams for haemorrhoids

Keeping hydrated *by drinking plenty of water is the best way of avoiding constipation while you are pregnant.*

CARPAL TUNNEL SYNDROME

The extra fluid retention of pregnancy can exacerbate a common condition known as carpal tunnel syndrome. Between 25 and 50 per cent of pregnant women will notice some symptoms of carpal tunnel syndrome.

This condition occurs because one of the nerves that supply sensation to the hand, the median nerve, has to pass through a very narrow space in the wrist, called the carpal tunnel, where the nerve enters your hand from your arm.

During pregnancy, even slight swelling in the hands can cause the nerve to become compressed as it goes though the carpal tunnel. Nerve compression is also likely to be worse the more weight you gain during pregnancy.

The most common symptoms are pain and numbness in the thumb, index and middle fingers and weakness in the muscle that moves your thumb. The main treatment of carpal tunnel syndrome during pregnancy is usually limited to simple things such as wearing a splint at night to help reduce pressure on the nerve that occurs when the wrist is bent. About 80 per cent of women will notice reduction in symptoms with splinting.

If you develop severe carpal tunnel syndrome, you may be referred to an orthopaedics specialist who may recommend steroid injections into the wrist to reduce swelling and inflammation.

However, most will not treat pregnant women as the condition will resolve. Do not take oral anti-inflammatory agents such as ibuprofen while pregnant, and try to avoid sleeping on your lower arms and hands. Symptoms usually improve within about 4 weeks of giving birth to your baby.

▶ **WHAT TO AVOID** Aspirin and nonsteroidal anti-inflammatory drugs such as ibuprofen

BACK PAIN

Back pain during pregnancy can be serious, and is one of the few problems that often persist after pregnancy. Roughly one half of pregnant women will experience some back pain during pregnancy, and the older you are the more likely you are to experience it. Carrying an extra 9kg (20lb) or more around your waist is hard on your back; each pregnancy puts a strain on your back and increases the chance that you will have persistent back pain.

The best way to protect your back is by keeping your abdominal muscles in shape before you get pregnant. During pregnancy, make sure that if you lift something heavy (such as your other children) you use your legs and not your back alone. Listen to your body, and

Back pain is particularly common in women over 35, and especially so if you've had back problems in the past.

stop lifting something if you feel strain in your back. Make sure your mattress is firm, giving your back good support while you sleep. If you have a soft mattress, consider slipping a firm board between your mattress and your bed base for extra support.

If you do strain your back, take up to 650mg of paracetamol, and try using a hot pack or ice pack on your back for 10 minutes (whichever works for you). If you have back pain that comes and goes, make sure you call your doctor because this can be a symptom of preterm labour. If you've had back pain before and

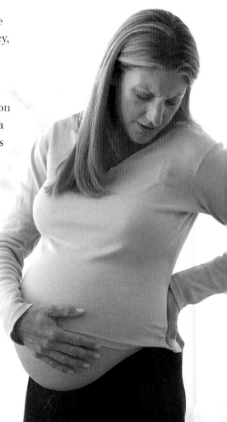

Safe Lifting

If at all possible, avoid lifting anything heavy, including your older toddler! If you do have to lift something, use the following technique.

- Stand with your feet hip distance apart.
- Bend from your hips and knees, keeping your back straight.
- Keeping the object close to your body, use the strong muscles of your legs to lift.
- Keep your back straight for the whole lift.

during pregnancy there's a strong chance that you'll have persistent back pain later.

▶ **WHAT'S SAFE TO USE** Paracetamol (650mg); heat or ice packs

▶ **WHAT TO AVOID** Aspirin, nonsteroidal anti-inflammatory drugs such as ibuprofen

SCIATICA

Sciatica refers to nerve pain that shoots rapidly from your buttocks down one of your legs, usually ending at your foot. Sciatica is caused either by one of the intervertebral discs (which lie between each vertebra) in your spine pressing on a point where the spinal nerve branches from the spinal cord, or by the uterus pressing on your sciatic nerve (which runs from the lower back down your leg). In addition to

pain, you may have other signs of nerve compression, including numbness or a "pins and needles" sensation in the affected leg. True sciatica is actually quite rare in pregnancy, affecting about 1 per cent of pregnancies. If you think you have sciatica, discuss the problem with your care provider.

SWOLLEN LEGS AND ANKLES

Most women at some point in pregnancy, notice swelling in their feet and lower legs. Usually the swelling is confined to the lower extremities. Swelling in your lower legs is made worse when you stand for long periods of time. If leg swelling starts to become a problem, try to take several breaks during the day where you lie down with your feet raised.

If you are working, try to move around frequently during the day. The action of your leg muscles helps return some of the excess fluid to other parts of your body.

If you notice that one leg is much more swollen than the other, notify your doctor because this can be a sign of a blood clot in your leg. However, remember that it is normal for the right leg to be slightly more swollen than the left because the uterus tilts in such a way as to compress the drainage of blood from your right leg more than your left.

▶ **WHAT TO AVOID** Diuretics are not safe to take in pregnancy

LEG CRAMPS

Some women find that they are awakened at night with sudden leg cramps. It's not clear why these cramps become more common during pregnancy. Calcium supplementation may reduce symptoms and is safe during pregnancy. If leg cramps make you wake up at night, try to walk off the pain or place a warm compress on your calf.

If you have persistent cramps, try to pay special attention to your calves before going to bed. Stretch them out gently by stepping up onto a step and pressing your heels down, one at a time. If you still have problems, talk to your doctor about magnesium supplements. Do not take magnesium supplements without checking with your care provider first.

▶ **WHAT'S SAFE TO USE** Calcium supplementation of 1g twice a day for 2 weeks

RESTLESS LEGS SYNDROME

About 10–20 per cent of women will develop restless legs syndrome (RLS) during the second half of pregnancy. RLS usually occurs as you try to fall asleep. You might have tingling or other sensations in your lower legs, which gives you the overwhelming urge to move your legs around. However, moving your legs or walking around does not relieve RLS. If your sleep is becoming disrupted, talk to your care provider.

Sometimes this condition is associated with iron deficiency anaemia, so iron supplementation may help. It's best to avoid caffeinated drinks in the last half of the day because these may make symptoms worse.

▶ **WHAT'S SAFE TO USE** Iron supplements

▶ **WHAT TO AVOID** Caffeinated drinks

VARICOSE VEINS

The pressure of the growing uterus and consequent increased blood flow causes a notable increase in prominent veins in your upper and lower legs. As the pressure in your veins increases, weakness in certain areas of the veins can cause the sides to balloon out. These are varicose veins. They may also occur in your vulva.

Varicose veins are more common with second and third pregnancies, but many women have them in their first pregnancy as well. Whether you get varicose veins or not is mostly genetic. You may be able to reduce the size of enlarged veins in your legs by wearing good support stockings designed for pregnant women. However, many women find these stockings hot and uncomfortable and only of slight benefit in reducing the appearance of varicose veins. Lying down with your feet up several times during the day may also help. If your veins remain enlarged after your pregnancy, you

can consider one of several cosmetic options, including laser treatments, sclerotherapy and surgery. You should wait until after you have completed all your pregnancies to treat enlarged veins because they are likely to return in subsequent pregnancies.

STRETCH MARKS

About half of all pregnant women will get stretch marks during pregnancy. Stretch marks often occur on the abdomen, but can also develop on your breasts and bottom. They are caused by microtears that occur in the connective tissue in your skin as the skin stretches.

Despite the claims made by manufacturers of various creams, no cream will prevent you from getting stretch marks. However, you can slightly reduce your chances of stretch marks by limiting your weight gain during pregnancy to 11–16kg (25–35lb).

Stretch marks will fade over time, becoming faint and silvery. While you can't prevent stretch marks, you can have them treated after pregnancy. Laser therapy is one option that is gaining in popularity, but is not available on the NHS. Plan on waiting to treat stretch marks until after all your pregnancies because you are likely to develop more with each pregnancy. Treating stretch marks is considered cosmetic and is not covered by insurance.

SKIN CHANGES

During pregnancy your skin undergoes enormous changes. Starting early on in pregnancy there is a big increase in the blood supply to your skin, which is euphemistically referred to as the "glow of pregnancy".

Early in pregnancy, the most common skin change you may notice is an increase in acne as a result of hormone changes. It is safe to treat acne during pregnancy with creams and gels such as benzoyl peroxide, or, after consultation with a dermatologist, with antibiotic creams.

As you move into the early second trimester, you may start to notice that your skin is darkening. Pregnancy stimulates production of the pigment melanin. You may notice that pigmented areas of your body, including existing moles and your nipples, darken.

New areas of pigment may also appear as your pregnancy

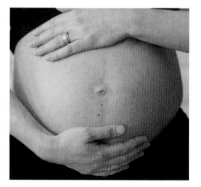

Linea nigra *is a common skin change of pregnancy. The dark line on the abdomen is caused by the body's production of more pigment during pregnancy.*

progresses, including a dark line between your belly button and pubic hair called linea nigra. Some women also develop pigmentation across the nose and cheeks. Both these areas of pigmentation should fade after your pregnancy.

About two-thirds of women with lighter skin notice that the palms of their hands turn red. This results from the increased levels of the hormone oestrogen in your body, and will disappear when you are no longer pregnant.

Increased blood flow to your skin during pregnancy can also cause the formation of tiny red bumps surrounded by little red lines. These blemishes are called spider angioma and occur most often on the face, neck, and upper chest but will fade after pregnancy.

No treatment is needed unless the spider angioma are still present 3 months after pregnancy and you don't like their appearance.

▶ **WHAT'S SAFE TO USE** Benzoyl peroxide (for acne)

SWEATING

Almost all pregnant women tend to feel warm during pregnancy. With this change in the way you perceive temperature and your increased metabolic rate, you are likely to notice that you are perspiring more. This is normal but can be irritating. Deodorant is safe during pregnancy so don't worry if you find you need to use it more frequently.

ITCHING AND RASHES

Many women have itchy skin during pregnancy, especially over their abdomen. Most of the itching seems to be associated with the skin stretching of pregnancy. Some women find that a cool sensation relieves some of the feeling of itching. Cool oatmeal baths or moisturizing lotion kept in the fridge may provide temporary relief.

Itching may also be a sign of a condition called cholestasis of pregnancy, which sometimes develops in the third trimester. It is diagnosed with a blood test that examines the level of bile acids (produced by your liver) in your blood. If your doctor diagnoses this condition you will be given medication to reduce the excess bile acids. The usual treatment is a drug called ursodeoxycholic acid. High levels of bile acids can increase the chances of complications in your current pregnancy and may prompt your

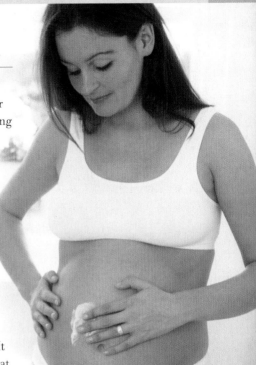

Moisturizing creams can help soothe itchy skin in pregnancy. Try keeping the moisturizer in the fridge so that it is really cooling to the skin.

doctor to induce your labour prior to your due date. It is not known whether treatment with agents such as ursodeoxycholic acid reduce the likelihood of pregnancy complications.

Warning Signs

If itching is accompanied by any of the following you should see your doctor.

■ A significant bumpy rash on your abdomen – this may be a condition called PUPPP, which is specific to pregnancy and needs more intensive treatment with prescription drugs.

■ Persistent severe itching on your arms and legs without a noticeable rash in the third trimester of pregnancy. This may be a symptom of a condition called cholestasis of pregnancy where bile acids from your liver build up in your skin, causing itching.

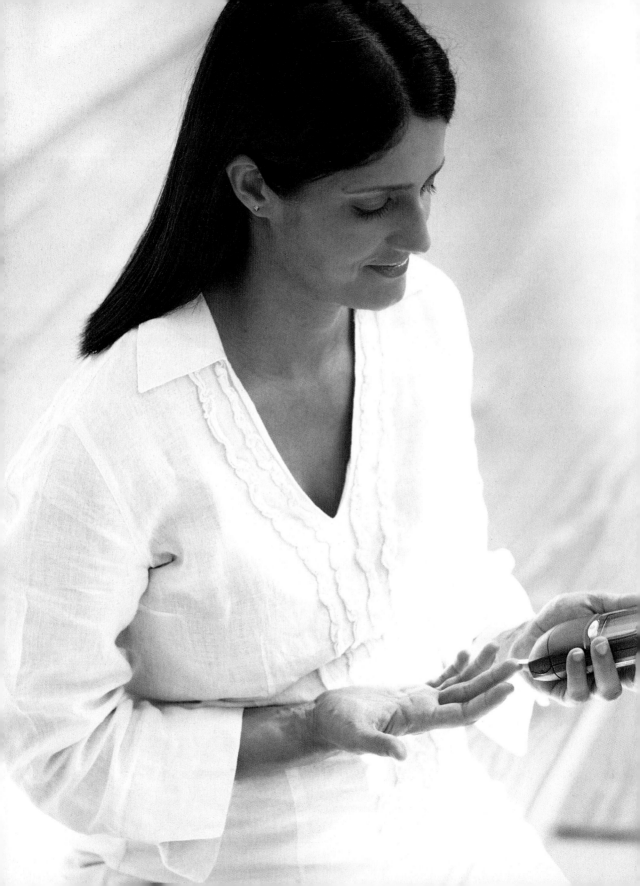

HIGH–RISK PREGNANCIES

Certain conditions put your pregnancy at risk, but these are not common and are not necessarily a reflection of your age. Many of these can't be avoided, but you can learn how to cope with them.

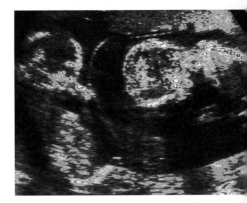

Twin pregnancies are treated as high-risk pregnancies needing extra monitoring. This coloured ultrasound scan shows the round head of one baby on the left, with its body below. The second twin on the right has its head facing down and body horizontal.

INFLUENCE OF AGE

As you enter into the late second and third trimesters of pregnancy, your age will play a factor in your pregnancy in a few key areas, placing you at (slightly) higher risk of complications.

The three most common age-related complications in later pregnancy are gestational diabetes, preeclampsia (toxaemia), and multiple gestations (twins or triplets). Some pregnancy complications are less likely to be related to your age – for example, preterm labour and cervical incompetence or insufficiency (in which the cervix opens too early.)

REDUCING RISK

In general, there is not much you can do during your pregnancy to reduce the rate of these problems. Your risk of preeclampsia, which is characterized by blood pressure and kidney problems, is closely

Checking blood sugar levels is key to looking after yourself if you develop diabetes during pregnancy, and will help make sure your baby is healthy.

related to your blood pressure at conception. The lower your blood pressure prior to pregnancy and early in your pregnancy, the less chance you will develop this condition. Gestational diabetes tends to run in families.

Both high blood pressure and gestational diabetes are more common in women whose weight is higher than their ideal body weight at conception; the risks increase as this baseline weight increases. Staying a healthy weight before you conceive will greatly reduce your chances of pregnancy complications, but not eliminate them completely.

Multiple pregnancies are also more common in older women, in part because of the increased use of assisted reproductive technologies. Women carrying twins and triplets are more likely to develop both preeclampsia and gestational diabetes. They are also more likely to go into labour early. While this list of possible problems sounds daunting, it is important to realize that most older women will not develop all or any of them.

Even though **you are over 35**, your pregnancy is **low risk** until **proven** otherwise!

types of high-risk pregnancy

Although your pregnancy won't be considered high risk just because you are over 35, your age does mean that you might be more likely to have or develop a problem that results in extra monitoring, tests, or treatments. Some conditions develop during your pregnancy, other conditions, such as high blood pressure, make your pregnancy high risk from the start.

GESTATIONAL DIABETES

Gestational diabetes is a disorder of sugar (glucose) regulation that occurs specifically in pregnancy. It means your body's ability to regulate your sugar levels is not up to the strain of pregnancy.

Normally, sugar levels are regulated by a balance between two hormones – insulin (produced in your pancreas) and glucagon (made by your liver). Insulin is released when your blood sugar

levels rise after eating, allowing your body to remove excess sugar from your bloodstream. Glucagon is released when your blood sugar levels are low, triggering a rise in your blood sugar levels.

TYPES OF DIABETES

In gestational diabetes, your body either fails to produce enough insulin to cope with the strain of pregnancy or your body's cells are resistant to insulin's action. This is similar to type 2 diabetes (sometimes called adult-onset

diabetes). Type 1 diabetes, which usually begins in childhood or adolescence is different in that the pancreas doesn't make any insulin at all.

During pregnancy, your placenta produces a hormone called human placental lactogen (HPL), which makes your blood sugar levels rise. As a result of this, your body has to produce more insulin to maintain normal sugar levels.

Gestational diabetes will disappear after your pregnancy is over, but you are much more likely to develop type 2 diabetes later.

HOW IS IT DIAGNOSED?

Gestational diabetes is initially detected in the third trimester of pregnancy by a random glucose test (see pp96–97) usually done at about 28 weeks. This is a screening test to identify women at a higher risk of sugar problems. Women who are found to be at risk of having gestational diabetes will then have a diagnostic test called a glucose tolerance test to determine whether or not they have gestational diabetes. Blood glucose levels are checked when

Diabetes and Labour

Women with gestational diabetes requiring treatment are at increased risk of having a large baby – the risk depends partly on how well blood sugars are controlled during your pregnancy. If you have diabetes, your doctor will usually estimate your baby's birth weight before you go into labour, either by feeling your baby through the uterus or using ultrasound. If your baby is normal size, your doctor may induce labour at 39 weeks because of the increased risk of fetal complications in prolonged

pregnancy in women with diabetes. During labour you need to have an IV (see p132), and your blood sugar will be carefully monitored every hour or two. If your baby weighs more than 4–4.5kg (9–9.5lb) there is a risk that the shoulders may get stuck (known as shoulder dystocia), which increases the chance of a birth injury or other serious complications. Your doctor will talk to you about this risk and may offer you a Caesarean delivery if he or she thinks you are particularly at risk.

you haven't eaten anything (fasting), then 1 and 2 hours after you drink a second sugar drink. If your blood sugar levels are high after your 2-hour glucose test, it means your body was not able to handle a sugar load and you have gestational diabetes.

Different care providers may use slightly different sets of criteria to diagnose gestational diabetes based on your blood test. Some doctors may consider a particular glucose tolerance test result borderline while others will want to actively monitor and treat you for the rest of the pregnancy.

HOW IS IT TREATED?

In most cases, gestational diabetes can be treated by adjusting your diet to reduce your carbohydrate intake. Your care provider may ask you to see a dietician who will advise you on what you can and cannot eat. You are likely to be told to eat unrefined, complex carbohydrates such as wholemeal bread, rice and pasta and avoid cakes, sodas, and sweets. Your care provider will monitor your blood sugar on your new diet. Your blood sugar may have to be tested up to four times a day at home, and you will be expected to do this testing

yourself using a simple hand-held glucose monitor. If your blood sugars remain high, you will need to have insulin injections (a twice per day injection) for the rest of the pregnancy.

FUTURE RISK OF DIABETES

If you develop gestational diabetes you are more likely to develop type 2 diabetes later in life. You should be tested for diabetes with a blood test or glucose tolerance test to check your blood sugar 6 weeks after delivery, and then at regular intervals after that.

CERVICAL INSUFFICIENCY

This is an uncommon condition, sometimes known as cervical incompetence, where the cervix opens (dilates) without you having contractions. Cervical insufficiency can be a cause of miscarriage in the second trimester.

If you have miscarried in the second trimester in the past – without having painful contractions – your care provider may recommend you have a cerclage in this pregnancy. This is a stitch that is placed around the cervix to keep it closed tight, rather like a drawstring around the neck of a balloon.

An alternative to a cerclage, in some cases, is for you to be monitored with a transvaginal ultrasound weekly or every other

week. A small ultrasound probe is inserted in the vagina and the cervix imaged on a screen.

If your cervix shows signs of opening up or of shortening, your care provider may recommend you have a cerclage at that point. Sometimes changes in your cervix

are noted during a routine second trimester ultrasound. In this case, if you've not had a miscarriage before, it is controversial whether placing a cerclage is helpful. Your care provider will review the risks and benefits with you or refer you to a specialist for consultation.

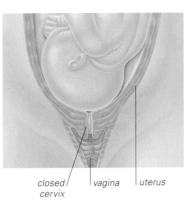

closed / cervix | vagina | uterus

The cervix is normally closed during pregnancy, except for a very small opening. This means that the baby is held securely in the uterus.

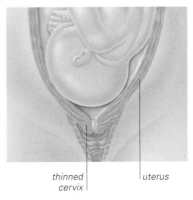

thinned cervix | uterus

With cervical incompetence or insufficiency the cervix becomes thinned and more open than normal, leaving a risk of a second trimester miscarriage.

PRETERM LABOUR

About 1 in 10 pregnancies result in preterm labour, where the baby is born more than 3 weeks before the due date. The chances of your baby being born prematurely are greater if you've had a premature baby before or if you are pregnant with twins or triplets.

Factors such as a higher socioeconomic status, access to good dental care (which prevents gum disease that causes inflammation), and not smoking mean you are less likely to deliver too early.

EFFECT OF AGE

Being over the age of 35 only slightly increases your risk of going into labour too soon. In some cases, this is because there's a medical reason for inducing you early – for example, if you have preeclampsia (see opposite). Women over 35 are also slightly more likely than younger women to have a condition that increases

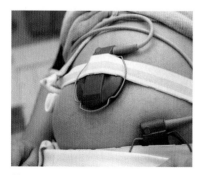

If your cervix is shortening or you are having abdominal pain, monitors will be used to check whether or not you are having contractions.

the risk of preterm labour. Fibroids (growths in the uterus) are more common in older women, and women with large fibroids may go into labour early simply because of the size of the fibroid.

Women over 35 are also more likely to be having twins, triplets, or more, either because of assisted reproductive technology (ART, see p29) or naturally, and this automatically places the woman at greater chance of preterm labour.

PREVENTING PRETERM DELIVERY

Unfortunately there is limited evidence to suggest that any drug treatment can prevent you from going into labour early. The results of a research trial has suggested that weekly progesterone injections decrease the risk of preterm delivery. However, the use of progesterone is still controversial, and progesterone injections are not widely used in the UK.

RECOGNIZING LABOUR

If you notice any repetitive tightening of your uterus more frequently than every 15 minutes, you should call your doctor or midwife immediately.

TREATMENT

If you are found to be in labour and you are less than 34 weeks pregnant, your doctor will usually treat you with medication (known as tocolytic drugs) to stop the labour. You will also be given steroids to reduce your baby's

chances of problems if he or she is born prematurely. Steroid treatment is most effective for your baby 48 hours after your initial treatment, so the first goal of treating preterm labour is to keep you pregnant for the first 2 days. You will be placed on bedrest and given tocolytic drugs. All these drugs can have side effects, so your doctor will usually stop your treatment after the first 48 hours.

MONITORING

After your initial treatment, your doctor may continue to monitor you in hospital or may send you home, depending on how much your cervix has dilated.

Fibronectin test Some doctors may use a test called fetal fibronectin to help determine whether your contractions are a serious cause for concern.

Preterm Labour Signs

Signs of preterm labour can include any of the following. If you experience these signs, you should call your care provider at once.

- Abdominal pain that comes and goes (contractions). If your contractions are more frequent than every 15 minutes or painful, call your care provider.
- Pelvic pressure.
- A significant increase in vaginal discharge.
- New onset diarrhoea.

A premature baby is likely to need special care. The risks to the baby depend on how early he or she is delivered.

have breathing problems or other complications and will need to be admitted to the neonatal intensive care unit (NICU).

If you are due to have your baby in a unit that cannot look after preterm babies, you may be transferred to another unit with better facilities for your baby.

PLACENTA PRAEVIA

This term means that your placenta is covering the baby's exit path – the cervix. Placenta praevia is often found early in pregnancy at ultrasound but resolves on its own in 95 per cent of cases by the third trimester. However, if your placenta remains in this position into the third trimester (past 24–28 weeks) you will need to have a Caesarean delivery to prevent serious bleeding. Until your placenta praevia goes away your care provider may want you to avoid placing anything in your vagina, which precludes having sex! If you bleed you may have to spend several weeks in hospital.

A negative test result means your chances of delivering in the next few weeks are low (1–5 per cent), and your doctor may then feel comfortable sending you home. A positive test means that your risks are higher, but it is still not certain that you will deliver immediately.

RISKS TO YOU

The potential risk of preterm delivery to you is low. You are more likely to have a Caesarean delivery because preterm babies often lie in a breech or transverse (sideways) position. You are more likely to have a uterine infection as this is one cause of preterm labour.

RISKS TO YOUR BABY

In contrast, preterm delivery can be very serious for your baby, depending on how early he or she is born. After 34 weeks gestation, the baby is at low risk of complications due to prematurity. If you go into labour after this time, steroids and medications to stop contractions are generally not given and delivery is allowed to go ahead.

Less than 28 weeks Before 28 weeks gestation, there are serious risks for the baby. One of the main problems is that the baby's lungs will not be fully mature and this can lead to breathing problems. Other risks include infection, bleeding from tiny blood vessels in the brain, and hearing problems.

Between 28 and 34 weeks The chances of long-term complications are substantially less after 28 weeks gestation. However, babies born between 28 and 34 weeks may still

PREECLAMPSIA

This condition, also sometimes called toxaemia, is a potentially serious form of high blood pressure. Women with mild forms of preeclampsia have blood pressures that begin to rise in the last few weeks of pregnancy. But unlike a simple rise in blood pressure, preeclampsia also affects other organs in your body, such as your kidneys and your placenta. Women with preeclampsia have extra protein in their urine, which can be detected by urine tests. No one knows what causes this condition to develop. There is no cure except for having your baby.

SYMPTOMS

Warning signs of preeclampsia in the third trimester include headache and swelling of the hands and face. If you notice unusual swelling or if you develop a new headache that is not relieved by paracetamol, you should see your care provider for a blood pressure check.

TREATMENT

If you develop preeclampsia close to your due date, your doctor will probably recommend immediate delivery. If you develop preeclampsia while your baby is premature, your care provider may place you on bed rest in hospital, to give your baby time to mature. You will be monitored for signs of worsening preeclampsia with frequent blood tests and blood pressure monitoring. Bed rest will lower your blood pressure and help your baby grow as much as possible.

Sometimes the condition becomes severe: blood pressure rises uncontrollably, blood tests may be abnormal, kidney function may be affected, and in some cases seizures (eclampsia) may occur. In such cases, immediate delivery is almost always recommended.

Since preeclampsia affects the placenta, some babies will not grow as well as they should and may not be able to tolerate labour. For this reason the chances of having a Caesarean delivery are greater than usual.

MULTIPLE PREGNANCY

As women get older, it becomes more common for them to have twins or triplets (or even more!). In part this is because the ovaries of older women sometimes release more than one egg per cycle. Older women are also more likely to become pregnant with the help of assisted reproductive technology (ART, see p29), which increases the chances of twins or triplets.

Although a multiple pregnancy can be an amazing gift, there is a higher risk to both the mother and the babies in these special situations, and all multiple gestations are carefully monitored.

TESTING FOR ABNORMALITIES

Multiple gestation complicates testing for genetic abnormalities early in pregnancy. First or second trimester serum screening for Down syndrome is considerably

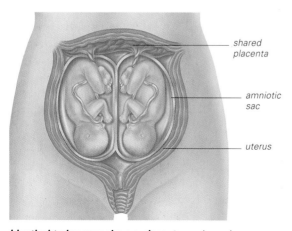

shared placenta

amniotic sac

uterus

Identical twins may share a placenta as shown here. The amniotic sac may be shared or separate.

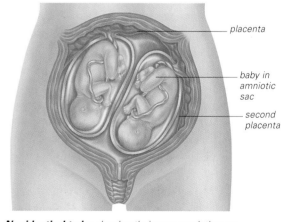

placenta

baby in amniotic sac

second placenta

Nonidentical twins develop their own amniotic sacs and have their own separate placentas.

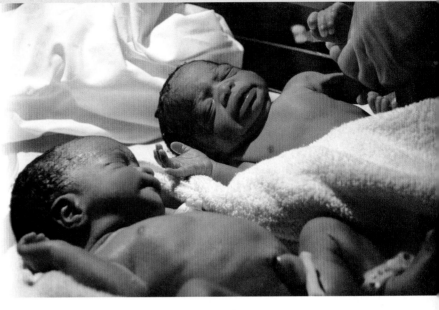

Twins may have to be delivered by Caesarean section. They will be carefully checked as soon as they are born.

less accurate in twins, and cannot be used at all in triplet pregnancies. Many women decide either to forgo testing or go directly to conclusive testing by chorionic villus sampling (see pp58–59) or amniocentesis (see pp80–81). There are further complications in testing twins. If an abormality is found in only one of the two babies difficult decisions must be made about continuing the pregnancy or taking the risk of reducing the pregnancy to a single baby.

RISKS TO THE MOTHER

With multiple pregnancies, there is a greater risk of preeclampsia (two to three times higher than with a singleton pregnancy), a slightly raised risk of gestational diabetes, and a 50 per cent higher rate of Caesarean delivery. For women who are pregnant with triplets, the risk of developing gestational diabetes soars, and almost all such women end up delivering by Caesarean.

Later in pregnancy, multiple gestation results in more maternal discomfort and weight gain – typically 16–20.5kg (35–45lb).

RISKS TO THE BABIES

Multiple gestation creates several risks for the babies, the main one being preterm labour. Half of twin pregnancies will have delivered by 1 month before their original due date, although the risk of very early preterm delivery (before 28 weeks) is low – approximately 4 to 5 per cent. Triplet pregnancies are at a much greater risk of preterm labour – almost all triplet pregnancies will deliver before 37 weeks and 12 per cent will deliver before 28 weeks.

As well as the risk of preterm delivery, twins and triplets are more likely to be growth restricted in the uterus than single babies. There is also a small chance that one may die around the time of birth. Although this risk is relatively low (less than 3 per cent), most doctors will monitor the babies frequently during the third trimester. This is done by regular ultrasound scans and heart rate monitoring (see p97), which check the babies' growth and well-being.

Most doctors also recommend delivery of twin pregnancies by 38–39 weeks.

LABOUR

The risk of Caesarean delivery increases with twins for several reasons. First, there is more chance that the first twin will be in a breech position (feet or bottom first). In these cases, Caesarean delivery is recommended. Second, placental problems and low birth weight in one or both of the twins are more likely, so they may not be able to tolerate labour.

If your first twin is in a head-down position, and the twins are about the same size, you should be able to try to have a vaginal delivery. Even if your second twin is in a feet-first position, a breech delivery can usually be quick and safe because the way has already been paved by the first twin. Most hospitals monitor each twin's heart rate separately throughout labour.

For triplet pregnancies, doctors usually recommend that the babies are delivered by Caesarean section.

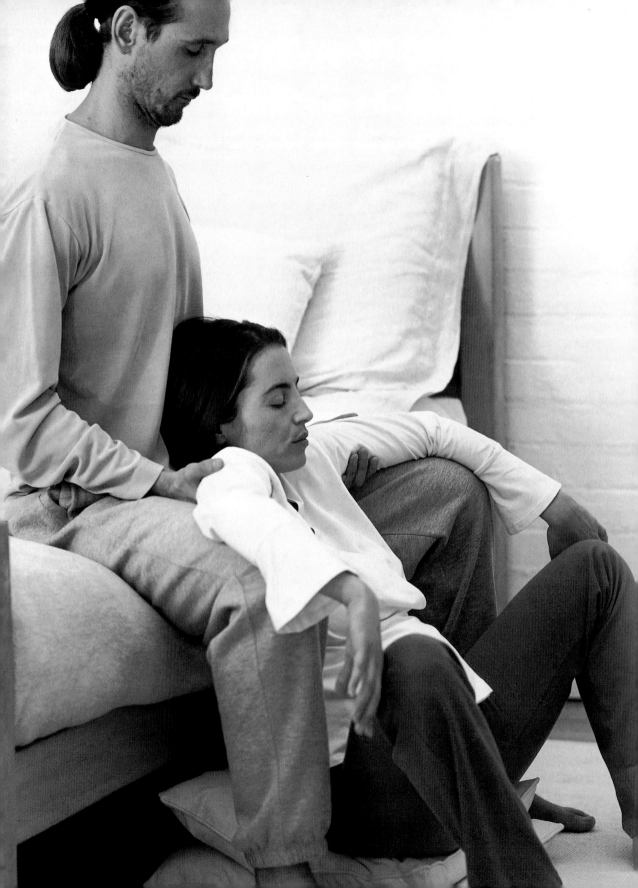

LABOUR AND BIRTH

Labour for most women is painful and exhausting. Sometimes it's easy to forget that this is what your pregnancy has been leading up to and that you are going to meet your baby for the first time.

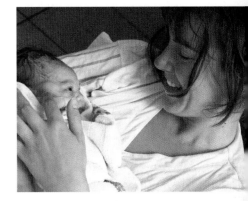

The joy of meeting your new baby makes the most prolonged and arduous labour worthwhile.

Labour is different for older women. Some of these differences are positive and wonderful. After the age of 35 you are more likely to be better educated about what will happen during labour and more likely to have an extensive support network. Knowledge and support are powerful, helping you participate more fully in health care decisions during labour, as well as ensuring you have support for the decisions that you make.

On the other hand, you may be more likely to enter labour with a medical complication where interventions such as electronic fetal monitoring are more likely, and you are at increased risk of having a Caesarean delivery.

COPING WITH LABOUR

As a woman over 35 you may be well informed about the various options for coping with the pain of labour. For first-time mums, it's hard to imagine what labour will be like, and there's a chance that you are more likely to get exhausted than when you were younger. Being informed of all the options for coping with the pain before you go into labour, from simple breathing techniques to epidurals, is really important.

Information-gathering is an important part of your preparations for labour, and you can incorporate your wishes into a carefully considered birth plan.

MEDICAL INTERVENTION

First-time mothers over the age of 35 are significantly more likely to have medical interventions during labour. These may range from electronic fetal monitoring to medications for speeding up of labour and Caesarean delivery. The reasons for a higher Caesarean rate in over 35s may be in part because more women are likely to have complications, such as previous surgery for fibroids, or placenta praevia (where the placenta blocks the cervical opening), that result in the need to avoid labour.

Being informed about possible interventions before labour and thinking about decisions you may have to make ahead of time will make you feel more in control.

Labour is **different** for older women. There are **benefits in maturity** and support, but drawbacks in what **your body** can handle.

preparing for labour

Giving birth can be scary for any woman. As a woman over 35, you may have already dealt with high-risk pregnancy care, and you may be aware of statistics indicating that older women and their babies often experience more complications during birth. Empower yourself with information and focus on the positive to help calm your nerves; give yourself the best birth experience possible!

Having to manage the uncertainties of birth is challenging for all women. Experiencing some degree of nervousness and even fear is normal. However, by facing your fears honestly, communicating with your birth attendant, and being prepared for the birth, you will be able to look ahead to this exciting event with confidence and relative tranquillity.

FACE YOUR FEARS

As the due date approaches, many women worry in particular about coping with pain and fatigue during their labour.

Coping with pain Giving birth does involve pain. For some women, this is one of the scariest aspects of delivery. However, the degree of pain you experience can be controlled in several ways (see pp126–131). Ask your care provider about the options available to you. Getting all the facts and understanding the different types of pain relief will help you feel more in control as you plan your birth.

Dealing with exhaustion More mature mums may be more likely to become exhausted during labour. Maintaining your energy is

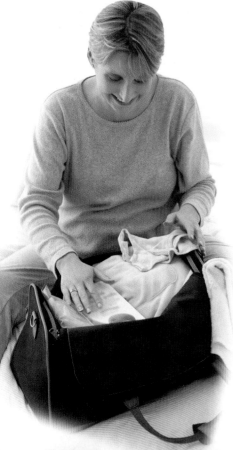

Pack your labour bag well in advance of your due date, so you can leave for the hospital at a moment's notice if necessary.

important, especially for pushing. If you are exhausted at the end of labour, your care provider may be more likely to recommend forceps or vacuum at delivery, increasing your risks. To help make sure that you begin labour with good physical reserves, get as much rest as possible in the weeks before your baby's due date and try snacking throughout the day so that you will not be famished, no matter when labour sets in.

BE PREPARED

Full-term healthy babies can arrive 3 weeks early. Having your nursery ready in plenty of time will reduce stress in case your baby comes before your due date. If time is at a premium, focus on the most essential nursery items first – your baby will need a place to sleep, nappies, wipes, and basic items of clothing. Everything else can be bought later. If you are planning a hospital birth, have your labour bag packed several weeks ahead of your due date.

If you already have older children, don't forget to make arrangements in advance for their

Packing List for Hospital

During your stay, the hospital will probably supply infant formula if you want to use it but the rest is up to you.

For your partner:
Necessary
- Small stash of cash for the telephone
- Pen

Optional but desirable
- Camera/video equipment
- Phone book of people to call
- Mobile phone or phone card
- Tape or CD player
- Massage lotion or oils; toiletries
- Snacks

For you:
Necessary
- Your birth plan
- Set of maternity clothes to go home in
- Hair tie for during labour
- Sports bra to bind breasts if you won't be breastfeeding
- Nursing bra if you are breastfeeding
- Toiletries and hairbrush
- Towels
- Sanitary towels

Optional but desirable
- Warm socks to wear while pushing
- Dextrose tablets

- Water bottle or sports drink
- Music you have chosen for tape or CD player
- Your own pillow
- Lip balm
- Nightgown/pyjamas/robe for wearing after baby is born
- Book on breastfeeding if you plan to breastfeed

For baby:
- Vest, babygrows, and nappies
- Before your baby goes home you will need a rear-facing car seat; an outfit for him or her to wear home; a baby blanket or shawl if cold

care when you go into labour. When serious contractions start, you'll feel more in control if you can easily contact your partner or other support person – and your midwife if you are having a home birth. Have a list of all the phone numbers you might need ready – including, if necessary, the person driving you to hospital or caring for your older children.

YOUR SUPPORT TEAM
Organizing good support for yourself can make a big difference, both emotionally and physically. There may be various people with you during your labour, each with their own supportive role.

Your partner or support person
The main role of your birth partner will be to help you remain

as comfortable as possible during labour. For example, he or she can hold your hand and rub your back, bring you a drink, or a fresh flannel to cool your forehead. Make sure your support person knows what to expect and what you want him or her to do before you go into labour.

Your midwife Your midwife will help manage your labour and keep you informed about your progress through labour. In a hospital setting your midwife will be available when you need her but probably won't stay with you the whole time. Your midwife will closely watch you and your baby to make sure that you are both doing well medically. She may be able to recommend various labour positions and her support can also

help to prevent you becoming exhausted and manage your labour pain better. Your midwife will teach you how to push when the time comes. Unless your labour is very short, you may have more than one midwife.

Your care provider Depending on the type of care provider you have chosen, he or she may or may not stay with you for much of the labour process. A midwife will be with you much of the time, whereas a doctor will check your progress intermittently and advise on interventions that may be needed to keep you on track.

When you come to deliver, your midwife will be there to guide you as you push. Your midwife may call on the help of a doctor if any complications arise.

your birth plan

A birth plan is a communication tool that helps you to clarify your preferences for yourself during labour and birth. It also enlists the cooperation of your partner or support person and your birth attendants in helping make your preferences a reality. For a birth plan to become a valuable resource, it needs to be realistic and endorsed by your healthcare provider. It should also be short and easy to read.

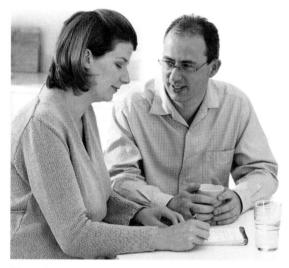

Discussing your preferences with your partner and writing them down will ensure that he understands your concerns and help him to act as your advocate during your labour and birth.

The first step in creating a useful birth plan is to become informed about the various procedures and options available to women in labour. It's also a good idea to become aware of the different approaches to birth, from home births to scheduled Caesarean deliveries, to see where you fit into the range of options.

WRITING YOUR BIRTH PLAN

To begin with, you may want to make a list of your most important desires for your birth experience. Typically, these include the type of birth you want – ranging from home birth to hospital birth, and who you would like to be present at your birth: your partner, relatives, friends, and/or your older children. You can then go on to list your most significant preferences for your birth experience (see opposite). Discuss your birth plan with your partner or support person and, if appropriate, with your midwife. Make sure they understand your concerns and preferences.

Contingency plans You also need to consider situations where the birth process does not proceed as expected. You should expect that your care provider will keep you informed about your options and include you in decision-making. However, in some cases, he or she will have to act quickly and the counselling and discussion phase may be significantly abbreviated. Make sure you are in the hands of a healthcare provider who has a similar approach to birth as you, someone you can trust to make optimal decisions for you in an emergency.

DISCUSS YOUR BIRTH PLAN

Near the beginning of your last trimester, bring your birth plan to one of your check-ups and ask your midwife or doctor to give you feedback. He or she knows about your individual health and the course of your pregnancy up to this point and can help you make realistic decisions that optimize the chances for a safe birth of your baby.

It is important to listen to the responses you receive, although, in some instances you may want to emphasise specific preferences, especially about episiotomy (see p135), so that your doctor or midwife understands what is important to you.

After your conference with your healthcare provider, you can prepare the final copy of your birth plan, incorporating all your care provider's input. It is important to make your birth plan as concise and easy-to-read as possible – ideally, the whole plan should be only one page.

Don't forget to make sure your name is clearly visible on the front page of your plan.

Make sure the right people receive a copy A copy of the final version of your birth plan goes into your healthcare provider's file, which should be handed to the staff at your hospital when you go into labour.

To ensure that a copy is available if normal information channels fail, it is also a good idea to carry a copy in your labour bag and give one to your partner or support person.

SAMPLE BIRTH PLAN

Name

Partner's name

Baby's name(s)

Other support person

Approved visitors during labour (always check with me first)

....

....

In labour I prefer:

☐ Intermittent fetal monitoring

☐ No IV

☐ IV OK, but no IV pole unless receiving medicine

☐ Labouring in various positions

☐ To drink beverages that I bring

☐ Amniotomy in active labour

☐ To allow my membranes to break on their own

☐ To labour in a bath or shower between checks of fetal heart rate

Please discuss any of the following interventions with me before they are done

☐ Oxytocin

☐ Amniotomy

☐ Fetal scalp electrode

☐ Uterine catheter

For pain control I prefer:

☐ Unmedicated labour, please do not offer me any medications unless I ask

☐ Opiates until I can have an epidural

☐ Entonox via a face mask

☐ Entonox via a mouthpiece

☐ Epidural when possible, but no opiates before an epidural

☐ Epidural as soon as possible

At delivery I prefer:

☐ No stirrups – my partner will hold my legs

☐ To try various pushing positions (side, hands and knees, squat bar, etc) to determine which is most effective for me

☐ To avoid a forceps delivery

☐ To avoid a vacuum delivery

☐ No episiotomy (please do not perform without my consent)

☐ Perineal lubricants (olive oil or glycerine, I will supply)

☐ My partner to cut the umbilical cord

☐ Place the baby directly on my chest unless there is a problem

☐ Check my baby and dry him or her off before placing on my chest

☐ I would like to see my baby, but please do not give him or her to me until my delivery is over (placenta delivered, any tears repaired)

After I deliver:

☐ I plan to breastfeed

☐ I would like to breastfeed immediately after delivery

☐ Please do not feed my baby supplements

☐ I plan to bottle-feed

☐ I would like the baby to stay in the room with me at all times

bringing on labour

The signals that cause labour to start are not well understood, but signs from your baby that indicate to your uterus that he or she is ready to be born are probably involved. Once your uterus is ready to go into labour, many other signals can stimulate contractions. However, if your body is not ready, things you try to start labour may only cause an increase in mild contractions.

HOME STRATEGIES

Probably the most enjoyable way to bring on labour is to make love with your partner. Human sperm contains natural prostaglandins that are a great stimulant to the uterus. Having sex is not harmful to your baby unless your doctor has specifically told you to refrain from intercourse for a medical reason. Stimulating your nipples either and other exercise that may cause a mild increase in uterine contractions, but are safe to try.

Herbal remedies These remedies are best avoided – some are potentially harmful, and the level of active ingredients within herbal preparations varies widely, so it is difficult to know how much medication you and your baby are

once your **baby** is ready **to be born** **signals are sent** to your uterus

during sex or by itself can also cause the release of oxytocin, a hormone that causes the uterus to contract and the cervix to ripen. This works best if the nipples are "rolled" between the thumb and forefinger for about 20 minutes. It's safe to do this several times a day. Other less effective methods of bringing on labour include walking

Walking won't necessarily bring on labour if you are not ready, but it can cause a mild stimulation to the uterus.

getting. Many powerful drugs that we currently use were originally purified from plants, and so-called natural preparations can still contain potent medications with side effects that can be every bit as serious as drugs you buy from a pharmacy. In the end, you must balance your beliefs against the scientific unknowns that surround herbal medicine. Castor oil and enemas are not particularly effective for bringing on labour and can dehydrate you.

MEDICAL INDUCTION

It is not surprising that many women beg to be induced once they approach their due date – or even before. After discussing your reasons with your care provider, choosing labour induction is an option, but there are risks. It is not recommended if you have previously had a Caesarean.

Risks of induced labour

Induced labour is less effective than spontaneous labour, and you are 1.5–2 times more likely to need a Caesarean delivery if this is your first baby. Induced labours are also longer than spontaneous labour, and you are likely to spend an extra day or two in hospital while your cervix is made ready for labour and contractions are induced with drugs.

METHODS OF INDUCTION

There are several medical methods of inducing labour.

Stripping the membranes This is the least invasive way for your care provider to stimulate labour. To "strip" or sweep the membranes, your provider will do a vaginal examination as usual and then run a finger between your cervix and the bag of water. This action stretches the cervix and releases natural substances that may help ripen your cervix and/or increase contractions. It is common to have vaginal spotting on your underwear afterwards, but you do not need to call your care provider unless the

---

Medical Reasons for Induction

Sometimes the medical balance is in favour of being artificially induced. In these cases, the risk of continued pregnancy to you and your baby outweigh the increased risk of Caesarean delivery. Some medical indications for induction include:

■ low levels of amniotic fluid in the uterus

■ preeclampsia (see p113)

■ your baby is not growing well (intrauterine growth restriction)

■ prolonged pregnancy (past 41–42 weeks).

---

bleeding is heavy, you think your waters have broken, your baby is not moving frequently, or you go into labour. Stripping your membranes will not increase your chance of Caesarean section. It only works if your cervix has started to open.

Cervical ripening Various medications or devices may be used to soften, thin, and dilate the cervix. Once the cervix is dilated and the membranes have been ruptured, oxytocin is usually given to start contractions (see below). Ripening is usually done with prostaglandins (administered as a suppository or gel) or with a Foley catheter (see p132).

A Foley catheter is a narrow tube with a balloon on its end, which is placed through the cervix while deflated, then inflated at the top of the cervix. Neither of these procedures are any more uncomfortable than a normal vaginal examination, but both can result in mild contractions.

Oxytocin This is a substance that is naturally released during labour.

In cases of induction, synthetic oxytocin is given through an intravenous drip to make uterine contractions stronger. It can also be used to strengthen contractions once you are in labour (see p134).

Some people believe oxytocin makes contractions unnaturally strong, but because some of the early painful contractions are strengthened, it may help move you more quickly into active labour.

Most hospitals will want you to have continuous fetal and uterine monitoring (see pp133–134) to check your baby for signs of stress if you are receiving oxytocin.

The amount of oxytocin you receive can be increased or reduced to give you appropriately spaced contractions.

Rupture of membranes If you have had a vaginal delivery in the past, and your cervical examination is "favourable", simply releasing the amniotic fluid from around your baby may be enough to send you into active labour (see p134). In some cases, rupturing the membranes may be done in combination with oxytocin.

labour over 35

The early stage of labour is followed by three distinct stages. Some evidence indicates that in older women who haven't had a baby before, the first stage of active labour can take longer than that of a younger first-time mother, but on the whole the principles of labour remain the same irrespective of maternal age.

EARLY LABOUR

During early labour, which can be short or last for several days, your body readies itself for the main event. You may notice an increase in "Braxton Hicks" or practice contractions. The muscle cells in your uterus are getting ready to act together to create strong, organized contractions. At the same time, your cervix is remodelling itself from a firm, inflexible protective gate to become softer and more stretchy. You may notice the loss of your mucous plug as the cervix thins out and opens slightly.

When to go to hospital If your pregnancy is low risk, you are almost certain to be more comfortable at home in early labour. However, you should call your care provider and/or go to hospital immediately if:

- you have regular contractions every 2 to 4 minutes that are so strong you cannot talk during them
- you have vaginal bleeding that is more than just a little pink on the toilet paper
- you have a gush of fluid from your vagina
- your baby is not moving.

Having one of your supporters rub your back can be a great help when coping with labour pain.

Stages of Labour

Active labour can be divided into three distinct stages.

■ **First stage:** This is the time when the neck of the uterus, or cervix, opens up to let the baby through. It is the longest part of labour – particularly in a first pregnancy.

■ **Second stage:** The cervix is now fully opened and the baby is moving down the birth canal towards the vagina and the outside world beyond. During the second stage you are pushing your baby out. On average, your second stage is longer during a first delivery than in subsequent ones.

■ **Third stage:** The baby is now born, but you still need to deliver the placenta. Your care provider will help by massaging your uterus and pulling gently on the umbilical cord. Usually the placenta takes between 5 and 10 minutes to deliver, but the process can take up to 30 minutes.

If your pregnancy is high risk, your baby is not head down, you have had a prior Caesarean delivery, or if your baby is growth restricted, you should go to hospital if you have regular contractions, even if they are not painful.

GETTING TO HOSPITAL

Do not drive yourself to hospital if you can possibly avoid it. When you get there, you will get checked in and the midwives will either put you directly into a labour room if you look like you are in active labour, or into an assessment bed if they are not sure. A midwife will take your vital signs (your temperature and pulse) and check your cervix. She may also monitor your baby.

If you are in established labour, your midwife may talk to you about your birthplan. If you are still in early labour, you may be sent home. This does not mean that you were silly to go to hospital – it is important for your care providers to know where you are in the labour process and to make sure your baby is doing well.

ACTIVE LABOUR

Every woman is different and enters active labour at a different point. Traditionally, care providers call labour active when a woman's cervix is around 4cm dilated. Most women are in considerable pain by the time they enter active labour, and are having regular strong contractions every 2 to 3 minutes. During active labour, your cervix should open at a minimum of 1cm per hour. If your cervix does not change as much as expected, there are two possible explanations:

■ your contractions are not strong enough, or

■ your baby is not coming down the labour canal to place pressure on your cervix and affect change.

Later in active labour, you may feel the urge to push or bear down as the baby's head starts to descend.

PUSHING AND DELIVERY

Your doctor or midwife will ask you not to push until your cervix is fully dilated (10cm) and out of the way. Pushing against a cervix that is not yet fully open can cause

tears and bleeding. When your cervix is fully dilated, you can begin to push. Usually your midwife will teach you how to do this. In many cases you can feel an urge to push even with an epidural in place, if your dose is reduced. There are many different ways to push, including on your back, squatting, on your side, and on your hands and knees. Pushing is hard work, and with a first baby it can take up to 2 hours without and up to 3 hours with epidural analgesia. Lots of emotional support is key.

DELIVERING THE PLACENTA

The last stage of labour involves delivering your placenta. The placenta is soft and squishy and easy to deliver compared to a baby. In most cases, the placenta will start to separate from your uterus and be delivered within half an hour of your baby being born.

Finally, your care provider will need to repair any tears that happened during the delivery, and make sure that any bleeding has stopped.

dealing with labour pain

Most women are apprehensive about how they will handle labour pain. If this is your first baby it's very hard to imagine what it'll be like. The subject of labour pain and pain relief can be highly emotional. You may want to avoid all possible medical pain relief, and with support some women find they do manage, but many more need help.

It is difficult to make a plan about how you want to handle your pain until you are having it. Every woman experiences pain differently, and you can't predict how you are going to cope with labour pain. If you start out wanting to avoid pain medication during labour and end up using pain relief, don't feel guilty or disappointed in yourself. You would never choose to have your appendix removed without anaesthesia, and this does not make you weak or a failure. Vaginal delivery is a very natural accomplishment regardless of the pain control you choose.

At the same time, it is unfair for your care team to assume that you will eventually decide on epidural analgesia and refuse to support you through unmedicated labour. You need to be prepared to stand up for yourself and your freedom to make an individual and guilt-free choice.

CHOOSING UNMEDICATED LABOUR

If you feel strongly about avoiding medication during labour, it is important to plan carefully.

Most care providers will be flexible and unlikely to impose their beliefs on you. The most important things to consider when you choose pain medication are the effectiveness of pain relief balanced against the side effects for you and your baby. (See pp128–131 for information on having an epidural and other ways of managing pain in labour.) The most important factors in the

Gentle lower back massage can help relax you, especially when you are in early labour.

success of your plan are your own knowledge base and the support of your care team.

Learn as much as you can about different positions for early labour and for pushing. Finally, choose to deliver your baby in a hospital or birthing centre that supports unmedicated labour.

During your tour ask specific questions about labour positions, the use of baths or showers for relaxation and pain relief, and ask about the availability of labour aids such as birthing balls. Think about bringing different kinds of music, and remember to pack some snacks to keep up your strength and remain hydrated.

MOVEMENT, BREATHING, AND RELAXATION TECHNIQUES

During labour, try different positions to see what feels right to you. Move around if you can between contractions; when you have a contraction, lean on a bean bag or against your partner. Some women find circling their hips or getting into another position helps. Repetitive movements during labour can also be helpful. You may want to try rocking movements, arm movements, and hand squeezing.

Some women find music during labour soothing, while others find it distracting and annoying.

Concentrate on breathing slowly and deeply, but don't get over-zealous about sticking to particular breathing patterns, which can lead to hyperventilation. Vocalizing with grunts, moaning, or swearing

---

Support in Labour

Having good support during labour can make a difference in how well you manage to deal with labour pain. For example, some research suggests that using a doula as the primary labour coach (instead of a friend or partner) decreases the likelihood of having an epidural for pain relief or needing a Caesarean delivery.

A doula is an individual that is trained to help support or "coach" you during your labour or support you after your baby is born.

Doulas vary widely in their level of experience, their philosophy, and their training. In some cases, doula services can be costly. If you want to use a doula, find one who is knowledgeable and flexible, and with whom you are personally comfortable.

Since labour is an intense and intimate time, if you choose a doula you will want to spend some time and effort checking on qualifications and making sure that you are compatible. Rates charged by doulas vary widely.

---

can help manage pain. Don't let hospital staff try to make you feel guilty for being vocal during unmedicated labour.

Massage Your birth partner can massage your back between contractions, and you may find this relaxes you. You might want to bring aromatherapy oils with you, if you find them soothing.

WATER

Using a warm bath or shower during early labour is safe and does not increase the chances that you will develop an infection, whether or not your bag of water (amniotic sac) is already leaking. Bathing is relaxing, and increases satisfaction and a feeling of well-being. Some hospitals have birthing pools, which can be used for pain relief in labour. Opinions and practices vary in regard to delivering in water, although

many hospitals permit it. Warm baths generally keep pain from getting worse for a while (about half an hour in one study), but may not make much difference after this. Therefore, bathing may have a short-term effect in decreasing labour pain and can be helpful in early labour, promoting relaxation between contractions. Women who want a higher level of pain control, may find bathing is only a temporary aid.

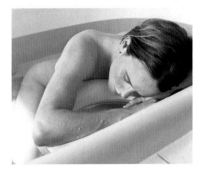

Bathing in warm water *can be particularly helpful in coping with pain early in labour.*

epidural analgesia

Many women find the pain of labour too intense to bear without effective pain relief, and epidural analgesia provides the best pain relief compared to all other methods. In the UK, more than 60 per cent of first-time mothers ultimately have an epidural. Many women have strong feelings about whether or not they want epidural analgesia, while others take a "wait-and-see" attitude.

HOW IT WORKS

Epidural analgesia works by delivering very small doses of an anaesthetic through a hollow tube to the epidural space, which surrounds your spinal cord. The anaesthetic numbs nerves from the waist down, including the uterus.

Epidurals are given by an anaesthetist. You will have to bend forward so that he or she can guide the hollow tube through a needle and into the correct position. You will have a local anaesthetic first, which may sting a little, but other than that you shouldn't feel any pain as the epidural is placed. Once the tube is in position, it is taped to your back to secure it so that more anaesthetic can be given easily at any time.

An epidural takes about 20 minutes to administer. Most women notice pain is reduced almost immediately, but the full effect may take 15 to 20 minutes.

The benefits of epidural analgesia are that pain control is excellent and that very little medication escapes into your blood-stream. This means that you are mentally alert, and your baby is not sleepy after birth from pain medication crossing your placenta. The other benefit of epidural analgesia is that medication is being given continuously, so you have pain relief for the entire duration of labour.

TYPES OF EPIDURAL

More modern epidurals, such as the so-called "mobile epidural", use the least amount of medication possible, allowing you to move

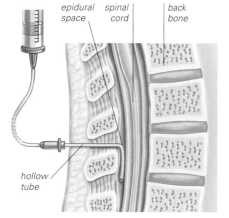

epidural space | spinal cord | back bone

hollow tube

An epidural is given through a hollow tube inserted into the space next to the spinal cord. The woman's back is curved to allow the anaesthetist to position the epidural correctly.

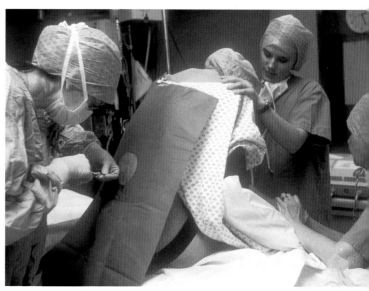

your legs and to feel pressure as the baby's head moves down the birth canal. Women who feel pressure can push more effectively, reducing the likelihood that they will need a Caesarean or forceps delivery.

Some hospitals allow you to control the epidural yourself by pressing a button that slowly releases more of the analgesic.

Another type is the combined spinal-epidural analgesia, in which a small amount of medication is injected into the space before the epidural is placed. This provides faster pain relief and is often used for women who are close to delivery when the epidural takes place, or when a Caesarean delivery is needed.

TIMING THE EPIDURAL
Many doctors will delay offering an epidural until you are 4cm dilated. However, this is an arbitrary cut-off, so if your pain is very intense, an early epidural is still an option. Discuss the various scenarios with your care provider before you go into labour.

SIDE EFFECTS
Like all medical interventions, epidural analgesia has side effects for you and for your baby, although the chance of a serious side effect is very small.

Longer labour Most studies of epidural analgesia suggest that contractions are weakened, which means there's more chance that

> ## Myths About Epidural Analgesia
>
> One of the big myths about epidural analgesia is that it is responsible for chronic back pain. But studies have found instead that pregnancy itself is responsible for back pain. Women who have back pain during pregnancy are more likely to have back pain after they have delivered. While you may have a sore spot and a small bruise on your back after epidural analgesia, choosing epidural analgesia does not place you at higher risk for long-term back pain.
>
> A second popular myth is that it will affect your ability to breastfeed. However, most studies have not found that epidural analgesia affects ultimate breastfeeding success.
>
> Your baby is much more likely to be sedated after large doses of narcotics given by injection (see p131), than from the small amount of narcotics used in epidural analgesia.

you will need oxytocin to return your contractions to their normal strength. On average, choosing epidural analgesia will prolong the active phase of labour by about one hour. Epidural analgesia can also prolong the pushing stage of labour by up to an hour. Since the pushing stage is often exhausting, an epidural can make it more likely that your care provider will suggest a forceps delivery (see p135).

Increased use of forceps
Epidural analgesia decreases your ability to push effectively, and approximately doubles the chances that you will have a forceps or vacuum-assisted delivery. Asking for your epidural analgesia to be turned down before you start to push may increase your chances of being able to push effectively and avoid a forceps delivery.

Fever Choosing epidural analgesia quadruples your risk of fever during labour. Although

most experts don't believe the fever is related to infection, you may end up being given antibiotics during labour. The longer you have the epidural, the more likely you are to have a fever.

Inadequate pain control About 9–15 per cent of women still have significant pain despite epidural analgesia. While this pain can sometimes be treated by giving additional medication, or replacing the epidural catheter, pain control cannot be achieved in all women.

Itching Up to 26 per cent of women with epidural analgesia will have itching, which is usually treated with IV medication.

Rare side effects There is a small risk that the anaesthetist may puncture the sac covering the spinal cord, causing spinal fluid to leak out. This can result in a severe headache that may be difficult to treat.

other types of pain relief

Although many women over 35 end up having an epidural to cope with the pain of labour, there are multiple other options. It's a good idea to be informed about these options and ask about them when you talk with your doctor or midwife. Types of pain relief range from complementary techniques like acupuncture to powerful narcotic drugs.

TENS

Transcutaneous Electrical Nerve Stimulation (TENS) works by passing a tiny electric current through the skin. This current is believed to block pain messages reaching your brain. It may also stimulate your brain to produce natural pain inhibitors, called endorphins. TENS devices are about the size of a small radio, and are connected to electrodes placed on the skin, usually on your lower back. Electrical impulses result in a tingling sensation, which some women find annoying. The side effects of TENS are usually no more than some skin irritation where the pads are stuck to your back. The electrical impulses do not affect your baby.

Most studies of TENS in labour have found it to be only mildly effective in reducing labour pain.

ACUPUNCTURE

Some women find acupuncture helpful in reducing labour pain. There are different theories as to how acupuncture works. In Western medicine, the hair-fine needles placed in the skin are believed to stimulate larger nerve fibres, which then block nerve activity in the smaller fibres that transmit pain sensations. It may also release endorphins, the body's natural painkillers. There is conflicting evidence on just how effective acupuncture is in reducing labour pain. However, it may somewhat reduce the chance that you will request epidural analgesia. If you feel strongly about avoiding an epidural, acupuncture may be helpful for you. However, you'll need to find a licensed practitioner who will be able to be with you during labour, and check the regulations at your hospital.

HYPNOSIS

There is some evidence that women who are susceptible to hypnosis may be able to reduce the sensation of pain in labour through hypnosis.

Hypnosis is a state of deep relaxation and concentration and is something that you can learn to do yourself (a technique known as auto-hypnosis).

While hypnosis is not harmful, it is expensive and only effective in women who are most susceptible to hypnosis. It may also only have

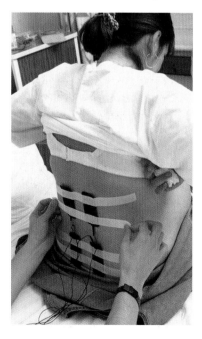

With TENS, electrode pads are taped to your lower back. The pads are connected to a device the size of a radio through which a small electric current is passed.

mild effects on labour pain. If you want to try this technique, you should start enquiring about classes early in pregnancy.

ENTONOX (INHALATION ANAESTHESIA)

Entonox is a mixture of nitrous oxide and oxygen that some women find gives good pain relief. Also know as "gas and air", entonox can be inhaled either through a mask or mouthpiece. It is only used during a contraction and although it sometimes makes women feel a bit "spaced out" the effects are very short-lived.

Entonox is particularly good at the end of the first stage of labour and while waiting for an epidural to become effective.

NARCOTIC ANALGESIA

Narcotic medications, such as pethidine and meptazinol, may be offered in labour. These drugs (also called opiates) are related to morphine and are given as an intramuscular injection. Narcotics slightly take the edge off the pain, but do not completely relieve it. They have the disadvantage of often causing drowsiness and nausea. Narcotics are most likely to be given in the first stage of labour before you feel the urge to push (most women tolerate pain better

once they reach the pushing stage and you also want to be at your most energetic and alert during this stage of labour).

Some women use only narcotics for labour pain, while others use this type of analgesia as a way to handle pain until they request epidural analgesia (which is frequently delayed until you are more than 4cm dilated). Narcotics affect your level of alertness, and this will take a while to wear off.

Choice of medication Most narcotic drugs are equally effective, and have similar side effects for you. However, some are possibly worse than others for your baby. Make sure you understand what medications you are being given during labour. Pethidine is commonly used in the UK, but this narcotic stays in your baby's system for much longer than other types, and causes more problems with alertness and breastfeeding. Meptazinol and morphine may be safer as they are eliminated more quickly. Ask about the options before you go into labour. Remember all narcotics have the potential to make your baby drowsy and affect the baby's heart rate patterns. If your baby is born sedated, he or she may be given an injection of naloxone to reverse the effects of narcotics you had during labour.

Since one of the side effects of narcotics is nausea, many care providers automatically give an anti-sickness drug with the narcotic. This may make you

drowsy. You can ask not be given anti-sickness medications unless you feel nauseous.

SPINAL BLOCK

Spinal analgesia is often used to block pain during a Caesarean delivery. Similar to an epidural (see p128), you will usually be numb to pain and light touch from the top of your belly down. Unlike epidural analgesia, a needle is placed into the spinal fluid (rather than outside the spinal sac), and a small amount of local anaesthetic is injected into the fluid. Leaking of spinal fluid occurs after about 1 per cent of spinals and can result in a bad headache. Spinal analgesia can't usually be topped up and lasts only 1–2 hours.

PUDENDAL ANAESTHESIA

If you don't have an epidural or if your epidural is not working well (a rare occurrence), you care provider may need to numb your pelvic area for a forceps delivery or to repair a tear. A pudendal block numbs sensation in the pudendal nerve, which supplies feeling to the genitals and inner thigh.

To place a pudendal block, your care provider will place his or her fingers inside your vagina to help guide the injection. A small amount of local anaesthetic is injected beneath the vaginal wall.

medical interventions

Sometimes birth isn't straightforward, and this is more likely to be the case the older you are. While many women carry an ideal of "natural childbirth" in their mind, the reality is that many medical interventions will be recommended to you in hospital. It is critical to think about these issues before labour since it is hard to take in new information while you are in pain.

INTRAVENOUS LINES

Some hospitals like you to have an intravenous line, known as a cannula, during your labour no matter what your age. It consists of a narrow plastic tube that is inserted into one of your veins in your hand or lower arm. Your IV does not need to be hooked up to a drip unless you are actively receiving medications or fluid through it. The tube can be kept from clotting with a small amount of anticoagulant, and the IV covered with plastic if you want to take a bath. An IV can have several purposes.

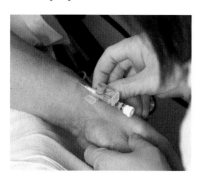

An intravenous (IV) line is placed in a vein in the lower arm or hand so that drugs and fluids can be given quickly.

■ It can be used to give you different medications, such as oxytocin for speeding up labour (see p134).
■ It can be used to make sure you have plenty of fluids (it's often hard to drink enough when you are in labour.) The drawback is that you have to be hooked up to a bag of fluid attached to an IV pole, making you less mobile.
■ Blood and medications can be given quickly if needed.

Pros and cons The risks of having an IV are very small, but an IV can be annoying. The benefits can be very real. For example, if you know you want epidural analgesia, you must have an IV. Keeping well hydrated (by intravenous fluids) may even help labour progress.

In a study where IV fluids were given more than usual, the risk of a long labour (more than 12 hours) was reduced by half. Last, while rare, profuse bleeding is a major cause of death during childbirth. An IV is an insurance policy that you can be treated quickly if the worst happens.

FOLEY CATHETER

A catheter is a tube that is placed in your bladder and attached to a bag that is used to collect your urine. A Foley catheter with a small balloon attached to the end is also sometimes used to bring on labour (see pp122–123).

If you have a Caesarean delivery, or a complication that can affect your kidneys – such as preeclampsia – then you'll need to have a catheter that's left in place around the time of your delivery to check how your kidneys are working.

However, in many situations you can avoid a catheter, and even if it is suggested when you have epidural analgesia, it is probably safer to try to use the bedpan. If you cannot urinate on your own, the nurse can place a catheter in your bladder every few hours, but remove it each time. The risk of bladder and kidney infection is less using either of these strategies than with a tube that stays in your bladder the whole time. Bladder infections can make you ill and prolong the length of time you need to stay in hospital.

MONITORING

During labour, you will be monitored regularly to confirm that your baby is coping with labour and to check your contractions. Electronic fetal monitoring (EFM) refers to the combination of devices that listen to your baby's heart rate and time your contractions. You may be offered either continuous or intermittent monitoring.

INTERMITTENT MONITORING

Unless your pregnancy is high risk (not based on your age alone), you do not need to be monitored all the time during labour. Studies have shown that intermittent monitoring is just as safe as continuous monitoring, provided that you have your own midwife. Your baby's heart rate will be checked every half hour during active labour, and every 15 minutes while you are pushing.

CONTINUOUS MONITORING

With continuous monitoring, your baby and your contractions are monitored almost all the time. However, in most cases, there is no reason why you cannot stand, sit or squat with the monitors in position. During EFM one or two elastic belts are placed around your abdomen to hold the monitors in place. One of these is a circular ultrasound-like device that checks the baby's heart rate; the second is a small plunger that monitors contractions.

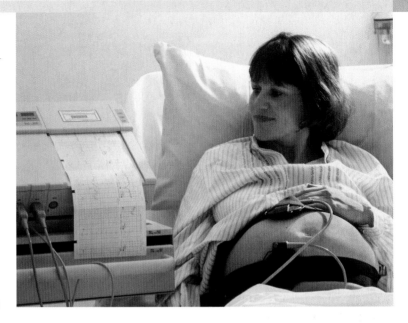

Some hospitals have monitoring equipment that allows you to walk around as much as you want and be monitored by radio signal.

Pros and cons With continuous electronic fetal monitoring you are more likely to end up having Caesarean delivery or a forceps (see p135) or vacuum-assisted (see p136) delivery. The reason is that your care provider may see changes in your baby's heart rate that are a cause for concern. Unfortunately, it is impossible to know the cause of many heart rate abnormalities – it may be something minor or it may indicate a fall in oxygen levels, which is potentially serious. No one wants to take any risks with your baby, so the doctors may recommend taking a sample of blood from the baby's scalp to see how he or she is coping with the labour. If the blood sample shows a low oxygen level, a Caesarean

The baby's heart rate and the strength of contractions can be monitored and recorded on a machine next to the bed.

may be recommended unless delivery is imminent.

If the fetal heart rate changes happen while you are pushing, your care provider may recommend a forceps or vacuum delivery. As well as increasing your risk of Caesarean, you may find the belts uncomfortable. The benefits of electronic fetal monitoring are not completely clear, although experts agree that continuous monitoring reduces the small chance that your baby will have a seizure after birth.

Most hospitals have policies that require you to have a minimum of intermittent fetal monitoring. You can refuse electronic monitoring if you feel strongly about this, and will be supported if your request is reasonable.

SCALP ELECTRODE

A scalp electrode is another way to electronically monitor your baby's heart rate. Instead of listening through your skin and uterus, a small wire is placed in your baby's scalp. The scalp electrode is placed during a vaginal examination and will not feel uncomfortable. It is used if your care provider is concerned about your baby's heart rate or cannot get a good signal using an external monitor.

Disadvantages The risks to your baby are small. There is a slight risk that your baby can get a scalp infection, which can be treated with antibiotics. Your doctor or midwife should discuss the scalp electrode first, and you should understand why it is being done.

Once a scalp electrode has been placed you cannot move far from the heart rate monitor, although you should be able to change labour positions. Some hospitals have radio monitors.

INTRAUTERINE CATHETER

An intrauterine catheter is used to better assess the intrauterine contractions. It is a thin flexible tube that is usually placed during a vaginal examination – it is not particularly painful, and you will probably not notice it after it is placed. Although the risks of a uterine catheter are low, they are not placed routinely.

You should be told when a uterine catheter is being placed and why it is being done.

SPEEDING UP LABOUR

If you are in active labour but your cervix is not continuing to dilate (open) as expected, your care provider may suggest your labour is speeded up (augmented) by one of two ways: breaking the amniotic membranes (amniotomy) or oxytocin. The chances of you needing this intervention is greater as you get older, especially if this is your first pregnancy.

AMNIOTOMY

Breaking the bag of waters (amniotomy) is painless and not likely to be harmful to you or your baby. It can shorten the time you are in labour by 1–2 hours. It can also significantly decrease the chance that you will need oxytocin (see below) in labour. However, it does not decrease the risk of Caesarean delivery.

In first-time mothers, breaking the waters is probably safest when it is done in active labour (after the cervix has dilated at least 4cm). If you have already had a vaginal delivery, amniotomy is safe at earlier stages, and can even be used to put you into labour. To release the amniotic fluid, your doctor or midwife will do a vaginal examination, during which he or she should be able to feel the bag of water through your cervix. Using a plastic instrument with a hooked end, a small hole will be made in the amniotic membrane, allowing the fluid to leak out.

OXYTOCIN

Oxytocin is a synthetic form of a natural substance released from your pituitary gland. Oxytocin is usually given during established labour because contractions are too infrequent or too weak for labour to "progress" effectively. (It is also used to induce labour, see p123.) Once you are in active labour (when the cervix has dilated to at least 4cm), most care providers like to see that the cervix is dilating by at least 1cm an hour.

Women over 35 are more likely to need oxytocin during labour to keep labour progressing. Once you start getting oxytocin, you must be hooked up to an IV pole. Some women worry that contractions will be too strong and too painful after oxytocin. One way to look at this is that weaker contractions aren't doing you much good. If you have to be in pain, it's better to have the pain be effective in dilating your cervix. You are more likely to need oxytocin after epidural analgesia, but in this case you won't feel the stronger contractions.

Oxytocin is usually started at a low dose and increased over a period of time. If contractions become too strong or too frequent, the dose can be turned down and the oxytocin quickly clears from your system. Used correctly, oxytocin is safe, and can reduce the chance that you will need a Caesarean delivery. Oxytocin is also commonly given after you have delivered to decrease vaginal bleeding and keep the uterus firm.

EPISIOTOMY

Episiotomy is a cut that your care provider makes at the vaginal opening to help deliver your baby more quickly. Episiotomy used to be performed routinely, but midwives and doctors now understand that tearing is not necessarily bad and episiotomy doesn't always prevent it. However, if your baby is in distress and needs to be delivered quickly, an episiotomy may be necessary.

In the UK, the cut is usually made towards the back of your right thigh (mediolateral). A midline episiotomy (where the cut is made towards the rectum) more than doubles the chance of a serious tear into the tissues surrounding your rectum or into the rectum itself. Mediolateral episiotomy does not increase the risk of rectal tearing but recovery can be more painful than when you tear on your own. Tearing into the rectal muscles or into the rectum doubles your chances of losing control of bowel movements, although this is still quite a small risk. Both of these problems are difficult to correct by surgery.

Given the potential long-term risks after episiotomy, it is in your best interest to talk seriously with your care provider early in pregnancy about this important topic. Most midwives and doctors only do episiotomies when the baby is in distress and needs to be delivered quickly. Episiotomies are repaired similarly to regular obstetric tears (see p136).

FORCEPS DELIVERY

Forceps are metal paddles that are used to guide the baby's head out from the vagina. In general, forceps are not harmful for your baby although birth injuries very rarely occur. However, the use of forceps does have substantial risks for you, increasing your chances of having a significant tear into the rectal muscles, especially if this is your first delivery. An extensive tear then increases your chances of incontinence of gas or stool (losing control of bowel movements).

The risk of a significant tear after forceps delivery is about 30 per cent in first-time mothers, although only a small proportion with a tear will have subsequent incontinence. Despite these risks, forceps may be needed if your baby has signs of distress at the end of labour – a forceps delivery can get your baby out much more quickly and, therefore, may be safer for your baby than a Caesarean. If forceps delivery is being offered to shorten the pushing stage, or because you are very tired, you may want to consider the risks. While some evidence suggests that pushing for a long time is associated with an increased risk of urinary incontinence, there is no good evidence that using forceps to shorten the amount of time you push reduces this risk. You have the option of continuing to push, or you can ask for a Caesarean delivery to prevent possible rectal damage. While some doctors may prefer you to have a forceps delivery to a Caesarean at this late stage, I believe the ultimate choice should be yours.

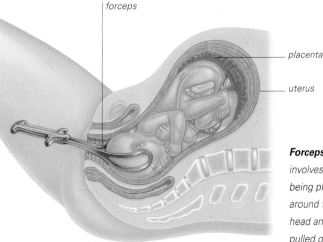

forceps

placenta

uterus

Forceps delivery
involves paddles being placed around the baby's head and the baby pulled out.

VACUUM DELIVERY

Vacuum deliveries use a plastic or metal cup that fits onto the back or top of the baby's head to guide the baby's head out of the vagina. The cup is attached to a tube that runs to a machine, which creates the vacuum.

Like forceps delivery, vacuum delivery is an effective means of delivering the baby if you become tired while pushing and the pushing stage becomes prolonged.

Since the cup uses vacuum suction to attach to the top of your baby's head, vacuum deliveries often cause scalp bruising. There is also a risk that you may end up having a serious tear. However, most evidence at present suggests the risk is somewhat less with vacuum delivery than it is with forceps delivery. The risk of injury to your baby is the same or slightly less with vacuum than with forceps delivery.

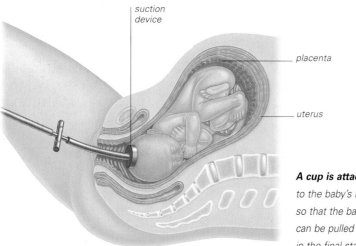

suction device

placenta

uterus

A cup is attached to the baby's head so that the baby can be pulled out in the final stage.

TEAR REPAIR

If you tear when your baby is born, your care provider will sew the laceration back up with stitches that absorb by themselves; no suture removal is needed.

If you have epidural analgesia, you should not feel much discomfort while this is done. If not, your care provider will inject

local anaesthetic into the area around your tear to numb it before placing the stitches.

After you deliver, your carer will show you how to wash the area and take care of your stitches. Salt baths are not necessary.

Usually your care provider will suggest that you hold off on sexual intercourse for at least 6 weeks so that your stitches can heal.

CAESAREAN DELIVERY

Caesarean delivery in labour is usually recommended if your labour is not progressing or if there are signs of your baby becoming stressed. Women over 35 are 2–3 times more likely than younger women to have a Caesarean delivery. If this is your first pregnancy, your risk of a Caesarean is around 30–40 per cent if you are in your mid to late 30s or older. If you have had a previous vaginal birth, your chance of a Caesarean is about 20 per cent.

A Caesarean section is a surgical procedure so if a midwife was caring for you, an obstetrician will need to become involved. Your partner or other support person should be able to come into the operating room and sit with you during the procedure unless you have a general anaesthetic.

ANAESTHESIA

For most Caesarean deliveries, you will be awake during the procedure but numb from the top of your abdomen down. This is achieved with spinal or epidural analgesia (see pp128–129). Although you are numb to pain, you will feel some pressure and the doctors touching you during the procedures; don't panic if you feel some sensations.

HOW IT IS DONE

The doctors usually make a side-to-side incision just above your pubic bone (bikini cut). Your abdominal

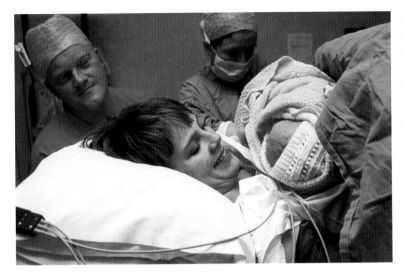

*A **Caesarean delivery** is usually very quick, and usually you see, and even hold, your baby soon afterwards.*

*A **Caesarean delivery** is usually very quick, and usually you see, and even hold, your baby soon afterwards.*

EMERGENCY CAESAREANS

If an emergency Caesarean delivery is needed, everything happens much faster. The important differences are that there may not be time for you to get spinal or epidural analgesia, and you may need to be put to sleep for the procedure. Another difference is that an up-and-down (vertical) cut is made on the skin since it may speed up delivery, although this is rare. Usually doctors will still make a side-to-side incision on the uterus. Occasionally, a vertical (classical) incision will be made if your baby is very premature and/or in an unusual position. Doctors usually avoid classical incisions as they are more likely to give way in subsequent pregnancies.

muscles are not cut, but are spread to the side. Next, the uterus is cut, usually also side to side. Your baby is delivered through the incision in your uterus and abdomen, the cord is cut, and your baby is handed over to your midwife.

You may have to wait until after the operation is over to hold your baby, but your partner should be able to hold the baby close to you shortly after birth. The time from the first incision to your baby being born is usually less than 10 minutes, especially if this is your first Caesarean delivery.

After your baby is born, the placenta is removed and the uterus is sewn back together using one or two layers of absorbable stitches. During this stage of the operation, it is common to feel nauseous or even to vomit.

Next, a second layer of stitches is placed in the tough material that holds your abdominal wall together, called the fascia. Finally,

your skin is closed using either absorbable stitches or staples. Putting everything back together usually takes 20–30 minutes.

If you have staples, these are usually removed 2–4 days after delivery, before you leave hospital. Having the staples removed is not painful, but feels like taking an earring out of your ear.

Ways to Avoid a Caesarean Delivery

Being older raises the chances of a Caesarean delivery. However, there are several things you can do to help reduce this.

■ Get into shape before you get pregnant. This will mean you are more likely to be able to cope with labour and be able to push effectively.

■ Avoid induction of labour if there is no medical reason.

■ Keep your pregnancy weight gain to below 35lb (16kg).

■ Drink plenty of fluids if you can during labour or have an intravenous line to keep you hydrated. This has been shown to shorten labour in many women.

■ Stay at home until you are in active labour – as long as your baby is moving well, your waters have not broken, and you are not bleeding.

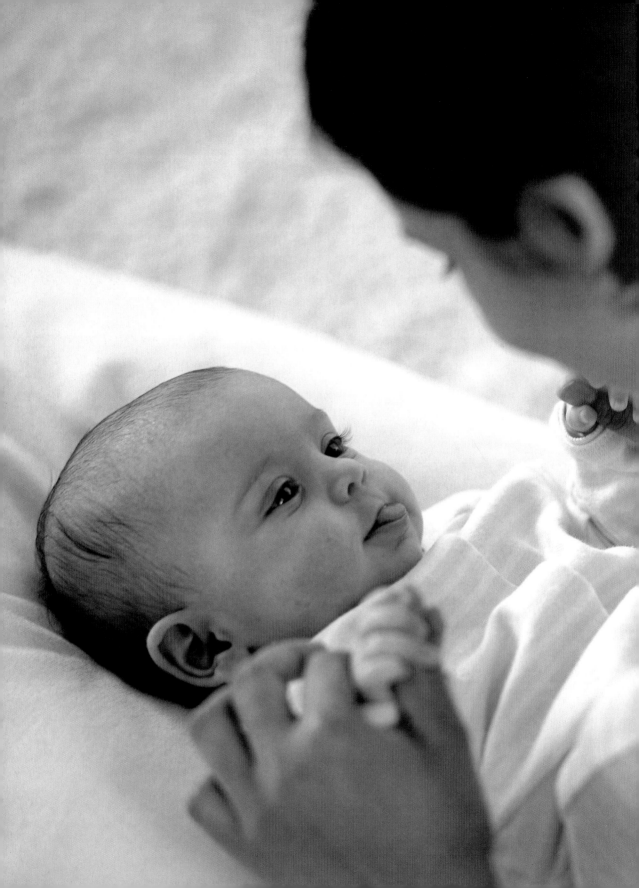

ADJUSTING TO MOTHERHOOD

IN **GIVING BIRTH** YOU'VE ACHIEVED SOMETHING QUITE **REMARKABLE**. NOW YOU HAVE TO ADJUST TO LOOKING AFTER YOUR **NEW BABY**. IF YOU ARE A NEW MOTHER, NOTHING CAN REALLY **PREPARE** YOU FOR THIS. YOUR TIME IS NO LONGER YOUR OWN, AND YOU MAY FEEL ANYTHING FROM **ELATION** TO **EXHAUSTION**, AND FREQUENTLY A MIXTURE OF THE TWO. YOU'LL **FIND SUPPORT** FROM FRIENDS, FAMILY, AND PROFESSIONALS IS VITAL AS YOU **FEED AND TAKE CARE** OF YOUR NEW BABY. YOU'LL NEED TIME FOR **YOUR BODY** TO RECOVER AND POSSIBLY PREPARE FOR **RETURNING TO WORK**.

post-labour recovery plan

Delivering your baby was hard work and the days following are often marked by a mixture of relief, joy, and exhaustion. Rest, diet, and exercise are all now key factors as you start your physical and emotional recovery. Looking after yourself in the days and weeks after the arrival of your baby will stand you in good stead for the months and years of parenting ahead.

Both you and your partner may want life to get back to normal as soon as possible after the arrival of your baby. However, it is important to listen to your body and not to place too great an expectation on yourself as you start your post-labour recovery.

GET ENOUGH REST

It's easy to underestimate how much mental and physical energy you have expended during the birth of your baby. Giving birth has caused major changes in your body, all initiated and controlled by huge hormonal adjustments. Getting enough rest facilitates the development of a new, healthy balance.

Your over-35 body needs more time to recover
There are several things you can do to provide your body with the rest it needs. First, even if you feel you have a lot to do, you need to take time to rest when you can. Try to catnap during the day to make up for lost sleep at night. Give yourself permission to nod off whenever you can, or at least lie down and relax. Second, accept help from family and friends. Acknowledge that you really do need to rest, even if you don't look or feel sick. For many independent women, receiving help from others can be difficult.

FOOD ESSENTIALS

Eating well right after the birth of your baby should meet several objectives. Your diet should help your body to heal, replenish physical resources depleted during delivery, and support your normal weight loss after delivery. Older women have often met with

some obstacles during the birth of their babies and therefore need to follow their healthcare provider's advice closely.

Continue antenatal supplements Most women should continue to take their antenatal supplements, at least for several weeks after the arrival of their babies. Breastfeeding uses up your iron stores so keep them up by eating iron-rich food.

Add iron-rich foods for energy Even a vaginal birth results in losing 300–500ml (about ¼ pint) of blood, and significant blood loss can cause decreased energy. Adding iron-rich foods to your diet can restore the oxygen-carrying capacity of your blood and with it your energy level. Good sources of iron include red meat, green leafy vegetables, and iron-enriched breads and cereals (see pp48–49).

Include vitamin C for wound healing Women with perineal tears, episiotomies or those who have undergone a Caesarean delivery all have significant local tissue damage. Vitamin C is helpful for optimal wound healing during the first weeks after birthing your baby. Vitamin C is abundantly available in fruits, vegetables, and in juices (see pp72–73).

Support natural weight loss Smaller, more frequent meals benefit your body's natural ability to shed some of the no-longer-needed pregnancy weight. Research indicates that women who don't lose their pregnancy weight within the first few

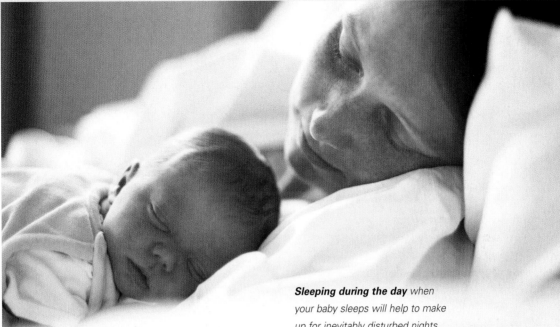

Sleeping during the day *when your baby sleeps will help to make up for inevitably disturbed nights.*

months after giving birth still carry that weight years later. This is an especially applicable consideration for mature mums who may have slower metabolisms.

Reward yourself with some comfort food The huge life change you are experiencing right now, combined with hormonal fluctuations, can make you crave your favourite comfort food. Often these emotionally soothing foods do not rank high on a nutritional scale. Making these foods a regular but modest component of your diet prevents bingeing in response to sudden cravings and encourages you to count them as part of your daily caloric intake. In this way, you can gently indulge but maintain control.

EXERCISE

Regular exercise can supplement your dietary efforts to support healing and, later, weight loss. Early in your recovery, however, you need to be gentle with yourself. Simply going for a walk is ideal for the first 6 weeks. Before starting any form of exercise, you should get your doctor's approval.

At all times, listen to your body and do not overexert yourself.

Yoga Yoga can be relaxing and invigorating, stretching and gently strengthening. It also can be done at home, near your sleeping baby. Gentle yoga moves can contribute to healing by providing oxygen to receptive tissues.

Pelvic floor exercises Kegel exercises strengthen your pelvic floor and may help resolve any lingering problems with minor urine loss. They involve repetitive tightening of the pelvic floor muscles. The easiest way to figure out how to tighten these muscles is to practise while passing urine. As you urinate, tighten your muscles to try to stop the flow. Once you know how to tighten your pelvic floor muscles, you can perform these exercises anywhere. Kegels won't do much if you do them infrequently, so try to keep at it.

Abdominal exercises In time, you will also want to focus on strengthening your abdominal muscles. Weak abdominal muscles often cause lower back pain, one of the most widespread ailments of otherwise healthy adults. Placing your feet on a chair while performing sit-ups or other abdominal exercises helps protect your pelvic floor.

early days

Being at home, as the main caretaker of your new baby, can be scary and tiring, especially if you are a first-time mum. Figuring out how bottle- or breastfeeding works, how to get your baby's arms through a shirtsleeve, or how to give a first bath can be challenging, particularly when you feel exhausted. You may need to ask for help with other chores, so you can focus on your baby and get some rest.

THE FIRST FEW DAYS AT HOME

Both you and your partner may feel uneasy caring for your baby at first. Your newborn may seem fragile and you may worry about doing something wrong. In addition, neither one of you may sleep particularly well because new babies do not sleep through the night. With all these changes in your daily rhythm, you may also wonder how you will manage going back to work in just a few weeks.

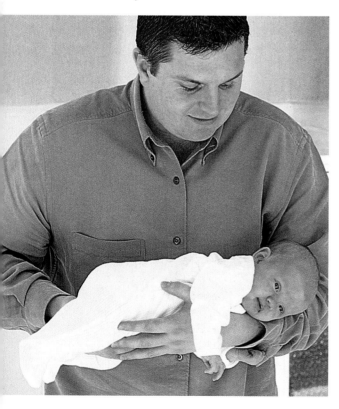

Realistic expectations It is important to realize that you will probably not have your life under control even several weeks from now. Being a parent is a messy business. Babies are unpredictable and with their arrival in our lives, they introduce an ever-present element of surprise. However, living with this unpredictability will become easier with practice.

Remember, babies are not as fragile as you may expect. Your baby just underwent a complete change in environment from a dark, cramped place to this bright, open world. With you close by, he or she can handle some parenting bloomers. Rest assured, your baby will whole-heartedly inform you when things don't go exactly the way he or she wants.

Accept that you will not be able to prevent all problems. Most mums worry about protecting their babies from nappy rashes, colic, and so on – and older mums may feel this even more if they have had a long wait to get pregnant or had a challenging pregnancy and birth. Take comfort in knowing that all parents have experienced this at some point. You will quickly learn how to handle things effectively, so don't feel guilty if you are not an instant baby expert.

JUST BABY AND YOU

In the early days, before you become attuned to your baby's more subtle signals, a lot of your actions may be stimulated by his or her crying. Communication is

Allow your partner to take over with babycare when he gets home from work. Laying your baby across your forearm and gently rocking him or her can help soothe intense crying.

simple for babies – if they are uncomfortable in any way, they cry. Crying can mean hunger, a wet nappy, or just plain fussiness. Try not to let your baby's crying make you resentful. It won't take long before you get better at deciphering why your baby is crying and fixing the problem quickly. Soon, the majority of your baby's time should be crying-free, unless he or she develops colic.

Remember that crying is not harmful for your baby. If you feel that you are becoming overwhelmed and angry, it's best to leave your baby safely in the cot and take a break for 5 minutes or so, then come back when you have calmed down.

DEALING WITH VISITORS

Visitors can help you feel supported and loved during the first weeks after the birth of your baby. A good conversation over a relaxing cup of tea can provide a wonderful escape from nappies and winding. However, it might be necessary to create some visiting boundaries that secure unstructured, restful time for you, as you get used to caring for your newborn while still recovering yourself.

During the first few days, you may just want to see your closest family and friends. Then, set some visiting hours – times when your baby usually sleeps, perhaps – so you can enjoy the time with your visitors.

it **won't take long** before you get better at deciphering why your baby is crying and **fixing the problem** quickly

Hold your baby when he or she is sleeping or happy In an attempt to create at least some time to get chores done in between feeds and nappy changes, it may be tempting to tiptoe out of your baby's room as soon as he or she is calm enough to let you go. However, it's important for you to spend some positive time with your baby. Have your newborn go to sleep on your chest, listen to music, and take time to savour being a mum.

Soothing a crying baby If your baby cries for more than a few minutes, even after you changed and fed him or her, pick your baby up. If your baby cries a lot, use a baby carrier to keep him or her with you. Most babies are soothed by being held close to your body (or your partner's). If this doesn't work, try taking your baby out for a walk or a drive in the car. Many babies are soothed by music or the sound of household appliances such as washing machines and vacuum cleaners.

Don't worry about over-pampering your baby. Calm, secure babies deal better with separation from their mums than anxious, lonely ones.

How to Beat the Baby Blues

During the first few days and weeks after the birth of their babies, many women feel very emotional and are often rather tearful. This is dubbed the baby blues. Try the following strategies to help. If these strategies don't help, talk to your care provider. You may be one of the 10–15 per cent of women who suffer from postnatal depression, a more serious condition that may need medical treatment.

- **Invite a friend to visit** Talking to someone who understands and listens can make all the difference.
- **Create time with your partner** Take the opportunities when they arise (when your baby sleeps, for example) to be alone with your partner.
- **Get out of the house alone** Ask your partner to babysit for an hour or two so you can get out and see your own friends or do something you enjoy.
- **Join a support group** Interacting with others who are in the same situation can make you feel better.
- **Pamper yourself** Take a relaxing shower and pamper yourself when you can.

feeding your baby

The decision to breastfeed or bottle-feed your baby can be an intensely emotional one. Breastfeeding your baby, even for a few weeks, can have some health benefits, but you should not feel like a bad mother if you decide not to breastfeed. Making the decision to breastfeed is a personal and private one; your individual situation may determine which option is preferable or even feasible.

BREASTFEEDING BASICS

Many women do try to breastfeed at least for the first few weeks. There are benefits for your baby if you can breastfeed – such as antibodies in breastmilk that help protect against diseases. It is also very convenient. However, if this is not what you want to do, or it doesn't work out even with support, don't feel guilty about bottle-feeding. Assuming you do want to breastfeed, be prepared for difficulties at first. You may think that breastfeeding is a natural process that you and your baby will know how to handle intuitively. Nothing is further from the truth. Correct techniques need to be learned, preferably from a trained lactation consultant or from another breastfeeding mum. Breastfeeding support groups can offer advice on any breastfeeding challenge you may encounter (see pp154–155).

What to expect right after birth In the last weeks of your pregnancy, your breasts naturally fill with colostrum, a watery-looking fluid rich in immune factors and beneficial proteins, perfect for your baby right after birth. On the second to fifth day after birth, your breasts will feel overfull and sometimes painfully hard. This signals the arrival of your true milk.

Latching on Learning how to position your baby's mouth properly around your nipple is essential for breastfeeding success. A good latch maintains your baby's continued interest in breastfeeding and helps prevent sore nipples. When your baby begins to search for your breast, use your finger to gently move down your baby's chin so that his or her mouth opens wide enough to accommodate much of the areola of your breast. Comfortable and effective latching on requires that most of your areola (the coloured circle around your nipple) be placed into your baby's mouth, not just the tip of the nipple!

Feeding frequency and milk supply Feeding on demand helps to ensure ample milk production. This

Choosing to Bottle-feed

Some women decide that breastfeeding isn't for them, or switch to bottle-feeding some way down the line. There are some important points to consider:

- Not all formulas taste the same. Your baby may prefer one formula over another.
- Buy only a few small bottles to start with and several kinds of teats. See which work best for you and your baby, then stock up with these.
- Clean bottles and teats effectively. Wash your hands before handling freshly clean bottles and teats.
- Prepare and use formula only as instructed by the manufacturer.
- Allow left-overs. Babies know when they have had enough.
- Feed more if your baby does not gain enough weight, urinates very little, and often cries between feeds.
- Feed less if your baby sicks up a lot when being winded.
- Don't change to more expensive hypoallergenic or soy formulas unless your health visitor or GP recommends it.

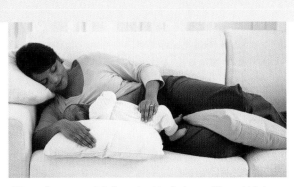

After a Caesarean it is important to find a position which is comfortable for feeding your baby without putting pressure on your sore tummy. Lying on your side helps in the early days.

may mean breastfeeding your baby as often as every 2 or 3 hours throughout the day for the first weeks. Short, frequent feeds will help to establish your milk supply. The goal for each feed should be 10 minutes at each breast, but your baby may not always cooperate. Try to coax your baby into staying awake by undressing him or her or scratching his or her back.

How to avoid sore nipples With frequent feeds, and nipples not yet adapted to breastfeeding, sore nipples are common during the first 2 weeks. Proper latch-on is the most potent protection against nipple soreness. In addition, removing your baby from your

breast correctly helps prevent nipple irritation. To do this, break the suction between your baby's mouth and your breast by carefully inserting your finger into the corner of your baby's mouth. Nipples can also become sore when they don't dry between feeds. Making sure that your breast pads and bra remain dry or opening the flap of your nursing bra to encourage air flow can help to prevent this problem.

When, despite all precautions, sore nipples do become part of your breastfeeding routine, keep a breast cream handy to alleviate your discomfort.

GETTING STARTED AFTER A CAESAREAN
Beginning to breastfeed your baby after surgery requires a little more determination on your part and support from those around you. Ask for a midwife to help you find a comfortable position for feeding your baby. Usually, you can lie on your side or, later on, be propped up enough to hold your baby in the clutch position (much like a little football under your arm). Since pain interferes with milk production and the let-down reflex, take enough pain medication to feel comfortable. Most pain medications given after birth, vaginal or Caesarean, are safe for breastfeeding mums and their babies.

Breastfeeding your newborn is a skill that can easily be learned with practice and perseverance.

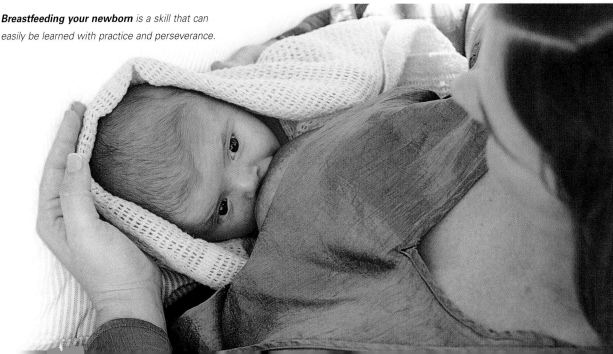

becoming a family

Introducing a new baby into your family changes the dynamics of your relationships with your partner and, if you have them, with your older children. Adjusting to a new baby can be difficult for everyone. Softening this transition as much as you can and working hard to set healthy patterns from the beginning creates the best chance of a healthy, positive family bond.

CHANGING FAMILY DYNAMICS

Life can be quite a juggling act for you when the new baby arrives, as you become accustomed to his or her routine and try and make it work with your family's existing routine. At the same time, you are recovering from the birth (see pp140–141). Your physical resources are low, so it's a good time to give your family new roles to help look after the baby. These roles are a challenge for everyone to adjust to, but in doing so, you create a wonderful family dynamic in which everyone is involved with the new baby. This is great for the new arrival, and also good for you because it gives you a much-needed rest at times.

Emotional Support

Many women work very hard to help their partners and children adjust to life with a new baby in the house. They may forget that the situation is also hard on themselves. Let your partner know there are many small ways in which he can support you during this challenging time. He can:

- Bring dinner home.
- Skip football in favour of watching your favourite film.
- Keep difficult visitors away, answer unwelcome phone calls, and discourage unsolicited advice.
- Surprise you with flowers.
- Tell you that you are beautiful (especially when you don't feel beautiful) and the greatest mum in the world.
- Put older kids to bed.
- Cuddle with you... and that's all.

INVOLVING YOUR PARTNER

Catering to the demands of a newborn all day, along with doing household chores, is exhausting work. You'll need a break from childcare during the evening to regain your strength. Ask your partner to leave the office on time and cut out weekend working so that he can take over the evening routine. Use the time to take a shower, read a book, or do anything that will help you wind down. Provide your partner with a list of things he can do to help you de-stress at the end of a tiring day. Most men accept a realistic to-do list, especially when it is given with an understanding that their efforts will be appreciated.

Comforting your baby as a couple Curiously, many babies have their daily crying spell just when their dads return from work. After making sure that your baby is not hungry, consider packing your crying baby into the car and going for a drive for 15 minutes or so with your partner. As your baby is lulled into sleep by the gentle motion of the car, the two of you will have the chance to talk after your long days, with no other distractions.

Helping him adjust to the new baby New dads can be even more intimidated by a fragile-looking newborn than first-time mums, but that is no excuse for them not jumping in and learning how to care for their baby. Especially for first-time mums, it can be gratifying to always be the first to soothe your baby and prove that you can do it better. Unless your baby needs to breastfeed try to resist this impulse. Your partner may never learn how to comfort your baby, leaving you effectively as a single parent from now on. Put in ear plugs, leave the room, do whatever you must to resist taking over!

In addition, dad needs to pick a few childcare tasks that are his responsibility. Being tired after a long day at work is an easy excuse for a reluctant partner; make sure he knows that you are just as tired. Consider asking him to be responsible for all nappy changing at night, dinner dishes, and/or baby laundry. If you have older children, ask him to look after the baby while you get some time with them.

A NEW ROLE FOR OLDER SIBLINGS

When a baby enters the family, siblings can become pressured to become the "older brother/sister" who helps to care for the little one. While they will slowly

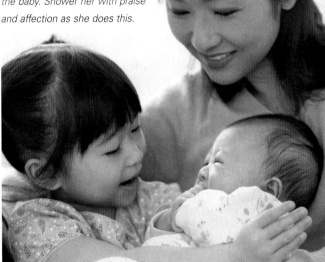

Ask your child to help you with the baby. Shower her with praise and affection as she does this.

seeing your other child or children with the new baby can be heartwarming. But don't expect the new relationship to be easy from the start

grow into this role, resist the impulse to force them to feel loving before they are ready. Children may worry that you love the new baby more – some jealousy and hostility are inevitable. Accept their feelings and reassure them that you still love them as much as you did before. If they feel secure, they will slowly come to see the new baby as belonging to them too.

Be patient with regression Seeing your toddler sucking his or her thumb and needing nappies after having been potty trained for months can be unnerving, but it's best if you indulge these needy ways. Such regressions are temporary and will cease once your toddler embraces his or her role as big brother or sister. A new toy or a special outing can make a big difference during the first days after the new baby moves in. Spend time alone with your toddler while your partner cares for the baby.

Give siblings a chance to shine Arrange for visitors to give attention to your older child. For example, you can tell them a great success story or a funny incident about the older sibling to divert admiration from the baby. Friends and family can be asked to bring something special for your older child.

Plan time with your teens Teenagers may not be enthusiastic about their parents having a new baby. They may worry about having to babysit and about not fitting into the new family dynamics. Often they withdraw, spending more time in their rooms or staying away at a friend's house. In blended families, teens know how families can change and may just not be ready to face another major family change. They need special attention during this often truly difficult time. Make an effort to cater to your teenager and make the time to spend with him or her alone.

a new world

As an independent woman you may find it hard to adjust to losing your freedom to your baby's need for round-the-clock care. Constant demands on your time will disrupt your life and may prompt feelings of isolation. A little strategic planning, persistence, and resourcefulness will open up a whole new world to you, one that is fun and stimulating for both you and your baby.

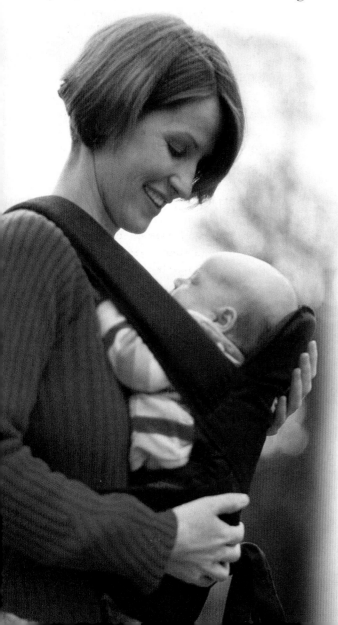

Baby carriers *are indispensable mobility tools. You can get on with chores as you are "hands-free," and get to places that are inaccessible with a pushchair, while keeping baby close to you.*

EXPLORING YOUR NEW WORLD

As you emerge from the safe cocoon of your first few weeks since the birth of your baby, you will want to broaden the scope of the activities you can enjoy with him or her. By now, you will probably be yearning for some mental, physical, and social stimulation for yourself, ideally in an environment that also nurtures your baby. It takes some creativity and exploration to discover the best new destinations that will offer you support and the best way to care for your baby when you are away from home.

take time to **find** some **new activities** you can **share** with **your baby**

Find family-friendly destinations There are mother-and-baby activities in most areas. Skim your local health club's listings for postnatal classes where you can take your baby, and look out for baby massage or baby gym classes. Spend time at a playground near your house, even before your baby can play on the equipment. The women who are there with their children can probably tell you about family-friendly recreational areas and activities, and you might make some new friends that you can share time with together with your children.

If you enjoy being outdoors, you may want to find some trails for you to walk with your baby in his or her pushchair. Consider safety and privacy for nappy changes or feeds.

Find helpful amenities You'll need to locate clean, comfortable places to care for your baby when you're out. In shopping centres and restaurants, ladies' toilets often provide changing tables. Good businesses also have pleasant seating areas where you can breastfeed. Dress-shop staff may allow you to breastfeed in a changing room, if you'd rather not breastfeed in public.

Restaurants often don't mind warming a bottle for an on-the-run feed – or you can order hot water or tea and ask for a large cup in which to warm a baby bottle.

Planning for your baby's needs The most enjoyable outings result from thoughtful planning that caters for the needs of both you and your baby. Some aspects of your baby's day cannot be disrupted without loud protest, so don't disrupt them! If your baby insists on an early afternoon nap of 2 hours, for example, try to accommodate it. You can stay at home during that time, have the baby in his or her car seat during a drive, or even go to a movie. You can engage in a variety of activities as long as they do not interrupt your baby's nap. With some practice, you will become proficient at predicting what works best.

A SUPPORT NETWORK

Meeting other new mothers can be especially rewarding as you bond over common ground. You can exchange tips on childcare, find out about recreational activities for young children, and get first-hand insights into local childcare options. Some women even form networks that exchange babysitting services with each other. To meet other mums and dads, go to playgrounds, mother-and-

baby gym groups, or parenting classes. You may be able to find details and meeting times for support groups in your local newspaper.

STAYING MOBILE

Having the most effective transportation for your baby will allow you to remain mobile. Invest time into finding the pushchair that works best for your lifestyle. If you like to speed walk or jog, consider an exercise pushchair. Make sure you have a baby carrier that allows you to run your errands efficiently and attend events with ease. A collapsible travel cot or playpen can provide the perfect place for your baby during visits at a friend's house. And a baby bag that accommodates all your baby supplies, is washable, and fits into your pushchair is indispensable for flexible daily schedules. Take some time to consider the myriad products for mums with active lifestyles. Good equipment can make a big difference.

Breastfeeding in Public

More and more women are choosing to breastfeed their babies in public places, and the more women that do the more accepted it becomes. Remember, as a breastfeeding mother, you usually have the law on your side if you choose to breastfeed in public. However, legal protection cannot shield you from the emotional insult created by those who are uncomfortable with your breastfeeding.

It is a good idea to make sure you are confident about breastfeeding before you first do so in a public place. Having someone with you – ideally, another breastfeeding mother – can be very reassuring.

Breastfeeding in public can be discreet, and often those sitting around you won't even notice you doing it, especially once you become adept at it. You can wear two-piece outfits to access your breast easily, and your baby can feed under the cover of your shirt. Alternatively, you can cover your breast with a nursing blanket. If you choose to breastfeed in public, try to project relaxation and confidence, rather than embarrassment.

going back to work

Returning to work after the birth of your baby can be both liberating and painful. On one level, you may long for daily contact with your associates and the faster pace of your work schedule. On another, you may find it difficult not to see your baby all day. Even though this divided feeling is strongest when you first go back to work, some of it will remain with you throughout the years to come.

You truly do have two jobs now – parenting and your previous career. And it is normal for most women to feel that, no matter which one of their jobs they are doing at the moment, they are neglecting the other. No amount of positive thinking will entirely eliminate a working mother's dilemma of trying to do it all. Try to do the best you can, and remember that children thrive on love rather than on perfection. Mums that stay at home full time are not perfect either.

ARRANGING CHILDCARE

It takes time to find an optimal childcare provider for your baby, and if you plan to return to work quickly after the arrival of your baby, you need to begin your search as soon as you can after he or she is born. Once your new arrangements are in place, plan to have some days before returning to work when you can drop off your baby for just a few hours. Most mums and babies handle change better if it comes in smaller increments.

With the right childcare your baby will thrive. It is important for you to feel confident about your choice, so that both you and your baby can adjust to this new arrangement.

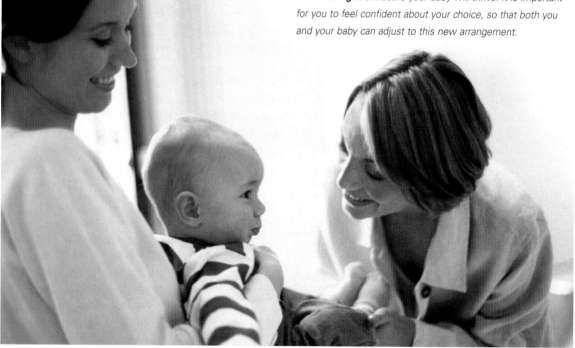

Locate a childcare provider For the most insightful advice about local childcare options, ask other working mums in your area. Then visit some of the places you are considering and stay a while to get a valid impression. Childminders, who look after children in their own homes, should be registered with the local council.

Have a plan for emergencies In addition to your regular childcare arrangement, you need to have a plan for when your baby is sick. Most nurseries ask you to keep your child at home if he or she has a fever, vomiting or diarrhoea. Therefore, you will need to either stay at home yourself or find a competent person who is available to help without much notice on those mornings that you cannot take your child to nursery.

Consider your partner's resources Your partner may be entitled to parental leave and may be able to stay home with your baby for a short time after you have returned to work. Remember that parental leave can be taken any time during the first five years of your baby's life. It also may be an option for you both to work part-time, so that at least one of you is at home with your baby.

Choosing a Nursery

When looking at a prospective nurseries for your child there are certain important considerations which you need to take into account.

- Does it have solid credentials? Recommendations from other mums are especially important.
- Is it clean and well-equipped?
- Are the caretakers interested and calm?
- Does it have an acceptable caretaker/child ratio?
- Is it in agreement with your childcare philosophy?
- Is it financially feasible?
- Is the location convenient (close to your work, if you intend to breastfeed)?
- Does it operate flexible drop-off and pick-up hours?

Employ a nanny Employing a nanny to look after your newborn provides one-on-one care for your baby in familiar surroundings. It also means you don't have to transport your baby each morning and evening and you don't have to worry about taking time off if your baby is sick. However, nannies can be expensive, and you should carefully check references and background.

MAKING THE TRANSITION

When you make your maternity leave plans early in your pregnancy, it is difficult to evaluate how you will feel about returning to work after your baby is born. A difficult pregnancy or complicated birth can change your physical and emotional well-being and necessitate a revision of your plans. If you feel this is the case for you, there are several solutions you could propose to your employer.

Flexihours Most employers will allow you to begin and end work earlier or later in the day. This flexibility may allow you to select a preferred nursery that opens later or closes earlier or to avoid rushing through your morning routine as you get yourself and your baby ready for the day. Sometimes, arrangements can be made to work longer hours for four days and then have an additional day off.

Telecommuting Your employer may be happy to allow you to finish some of your assignments at home. Consider splitting your workday into a half office and half home day. Alternatively, maybe you prefer to be at your place of work for two or three days per week and work at home for the remainder.

Work hours and benefit packages As you propose a more agreeable work arrangement to your employer, make sure you do not lose health insurance and other important benefits. You are often required to maintain a minimum number of weekly hours on the job to remain eligible for your company benefit package and it is essential to find out applicable requirements before you speak with your employer.

Becoming a Stay-at-Home Mum

Some new mums find that the birth of their baby has changed their priorities so much that they do not wish to return to their previous place of work. Mums over 35 may contemplate leaving careers they have built up for many years and need to evaluate carefully the consequences of this life-changing decision. Here are some points to consider.

Financial aspects

- Is living on one income at all feasible?
- Who would be in charge of financial decisions?
- Would you have access to your partner's income?
- How secure is your partner's income?
- Can you return to work if necessary?
- How will this affect your pension?

Relationship aspects

- Do you trust making yourself financially dependent on your partner?
- How is this change likely to affect the balance of power in your relationship?
- Does your partner admire full-time homemaking and motherhood?

Social aspects

- Would you miss the interaction with other adults at work?
- Will your friends and family support you in your decision?
- Is there anyone else at home during the day near you?

Career aspects

- Will you miss your work?
- Has your career been a significant aspect of your identity?
- Can you return to your career after several years of absence?
- Can you build your career from a home office?
- Are there educational opportunities for you during your childrearing years?
- Does it make sense to stay in touch with your employer?
- Is there a chance that you can work for your employer from home?

COMBINING WORK WITH BREASTFEEDING

An important consideration as the time approaches for you to return to work will be whether or not you want to continue breastfeeding and, if so, how this can be accommodated in your work place. Some employers provide support for breastfeeding, such as paid access to a lactation specialist, cost sharing for a high-quality breast pump, and the privacy of a designated breastfeeding room. Others will not consider your needs as a breastfeeding mum at all.

Breastfeeding gets easier with practice. As your maternity leave ends your breastfeeding should be well established, and it may be easier to continue, even under less than optimal circumstances. Although not ideal, supplementing your breastmilk with a small amount of formula at this point should not undermine continued breastfeeding.

Expressing milk at work In order to keep up your supply of milk and to prevent your breasts from becoming swollen, you will need to express your breast milk when you are away from your baby for any length of time. Effective breast pumps may be more expensive, but often allow you to spend less time expressing. Look for a full-size, automatic, electric pump with quiet operation, easy transportability, and the option to express both breasts at the same time. Usually, expressing three times per day will provide you with enough milk for your childcare provider's feeds the next day. Expressing frequently enough to maintain your milk supply can be difficult, especially if there is no comfortable, private place for doing it at your place of work, but if breastfeeding is important to you, don't give up on finding a solution that will make it work.

Coping with unexpected letdown Unfortunately, the letdown reflex does not only work when you intend to breastfeed your baby. It can kick in when you think about your baby or if you hear another baby crying. If this happens at work, reduce the visibility of leaks by using breast shields and by wearing layers or patterned tops, or by expressing more regularly.

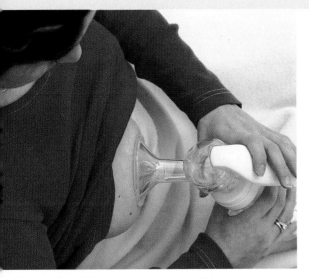

Expressing milk while you are at work will help you to maintain your milk supply and allow you to keep on breastfeeding your baby once you return to your job.

TIPS FOR SUCCESS

There are various measures you can take to help make breastfeeding and returning to work a successful combination.

Gain your employer's support Your employer may become more supportive of your breastfeeding needs if you can persuade him or her that your child will have less illness if you breastfeed. For example, breastfeeding is thought to prevent at least 1–2 ear infections and/or diarrhoea episodes per year. Therefore, you may be absent from work less frequently than parents of bottle-fed children, and a comparatively small investment from your company in your ability to breastfeed now may reap long-term productivity benefits.

Breastfeed your baby whenever you can
Sufficient milk production is ensured by a high frequency of feeds and your baby's sucking motion. Therefore, if your baby's nursery is near your place of work, you might want to try a visit at lunchtime and see if he or she is ready for a feed, although this may unsettle your baby. Otherwise, expressing will have a similar effect. You can also increase the frequency of your feeds before and after work. Most babies adjust their nursing schedules automatically, sleeping more while they are at nursery and feeding more when you are available. Also, take advantage of your time together when work has finished, especially the weekends, to boost your milk supply for the coming week.

Initiate the letdown reflex It can be difficult to focus on expressing breast milk straight after a business meeting or in the middle of a stressful task. You need to discuss with your employer whether or not there is a room where you can express in privacy. Ideally, you need a room with an electrical outlet and a locking door. Sometimes a phone call to your nursery or looking at a photo of your baby can help initiate your letdown reflex.

Store your breast milk safely Make sure that you wash your hands before expressing and that you use clean storage bottles to prevent the introduction of bacteria or viruses. Breast milk is easy to store. It stays fresh for 6–10 hours, even at room temperature. If you have access to a refrigerator at work, this is ideal for storage.

Breast milk can be kept for up to 3–5 days in a refrigerator and for up to 2 weeks in a freezer so long as you have a separate freezer compartment. Make sure you label each bottle containing fresh breast milk with the date on which it was expressed to avoid any confusion.

Supplement with formula If expressing does not work for you, don't feel you have to give up on breastfeeding after you return to your job. You may be able to breastfeed when you are with your baby and provide formula to your childcare provider when you are absent. (Formula is available in cartons, which may be more convenient than powder when you are working). Even if breast milk is only one component of your baby's diet, there may still be some health benefits for him or her and some emotional advantages for you, too.

resources

ARC (Antenatal Results and Choices)
73 Charlotte Street
London W1T 4PN
Tel: 020 7631 0285 (office hours)
www.arc-uk.org
Provides information and support to parents throughout the antenatal testing process

Association of Breastfeeding Mothers
PO Box 207
Bridgwater
TA6 7YT
Tel: 0870 401 7711
www.abm.me.uk
Information and support for breastfeeding mothers and their families

Association for Postnatal Illness
145 Dawes Road
London SW6 7EB
Tel: 020 7386 0868
www.apni.org
Advice on postnatal illness and depression

BLISS (Baby Life Support System)
68 South Lambeth Road (1st Floor)
London SW8 1RL
Tel: 020 7820 9471
www.bliss.org.uk
Support for parents of premature and special needs babies

Breastfeeding Network
PO Box 11126
Paisley
PA2 8YB
Tel: 0870 900 8787
www.breastfeedingnetwork.org.uk
Support and information for breastfeeding mothers

British Nutrition Foundation
High Holborn House
52–54 High Holborn
London WC1V 6RQ
Tel: 020 7404 6504
www.nutrition.org.uk
Promotes nutritional wellbeing

Eating for Pregnancy Helpline
The Centre for Pregnancy Nutrition
University of Sheffield
Tel: 0845 130 3646
www.shef.sc.uk/pregnancy_nutrition

Human Fertilization and Embryology Authority
21 Bloomsbury Street
London WC1B 3HF
Tel: 020 7291 8200
www.hfea.gov.uk
Government body that regulates and inspects all UK clinics providing IVF, donor insemination, or the storage of eggs, sperm, or embryos

Independent Midwives Association
1 The Great Quarry
Guildford
Surrey GU1 3XN
Tel: 01483 821104
www.independentmidwives.org.uk
Provides a list of independent midwives in the UK

Infertility Network UK
Charter House
43 St Leonards on Sea
Bexhill
East Sussex TN40 1JA
Tel: 08701 188088
www.infertilitynetworkuk.com
Advice and counselling on all aspects of fertility

LaLeche League
PO Box 29
West Bridgford
Nottingham
NG2 7NP
Tel: 0845 120 2918
www.laleche.org.uk
Helpline for breastfeeding advice and information

Maternity Alliance
Third Floor West
2–6 Northburgh Street
London EC1V 0AY
Tel: 020 7490 7638
www.maternityalliance.org.uk
*Advice and information about maternity
rights and benefits*

The Miscarriage Association
c/o Clayton Hospital
Northgate
Wakefield
West Yorkshire WF1 3JS
01924 200799
www.miscarriageassociation.org.uk
*Advice and information on a national network of
miscarriage support groups*

National Childbirth Trust
Alexandra House
Oldham Terrace
Acton
London W3 6NH
Tel: 0870 4448707
www.nctpregnancyandbabycare.com
*Information on antenatal classes and advice and
support during the antenatal and postnatal periods*

NHS Direct
Tel: 0845 4647 (24 hours)
www.nhsdirect.nhs.uk
Wide-ranging advice on health matters

Parentline Plus
520 Highgate Studios
53–79 Highgate Road
London NW5 1TL
Tel: 0808 800 2222
www.parentlineplus.org.uk
Support and information for parents

Relate
Herbert Gray College
Little Church Street
Rugby
Warwickshire CV21 3AP
Tel: 0845 456 1310
www.relate.org.uk
Offers family counselling and courses for parents

TAMBA (Twins and Multiple Birth Association)
2 The Willows
Gardner Road
Guildford
Surrey GU1 4PG
Tel: 0870 770 3305 Helpline: 0800 138 0509
www.tamba.org.uk
Support and information for families of twins and more

Vegetarian Society
Parkdale
Dunham Road
Altrincham
Cheshire WA14 4QG
Tel: 0161 925 2000
www.vegsoc.org
*Information on vegetarian diets during pregnancy
and for infants*

index

picture credits

The publisher would like to thank the following for their kind permission to reproduce their photographs:
ABBREVIATIONS KEY: a=above; b=below; c=centre; l=left; r=right; t=top.

1: Mother & Baby Picture Library/Ian Hooton; **2: Getty Images/**Nick Dolding; **7: Portrait Innovations/**Kate Cosby (bl); **13: Zefa Visual Media/**M. Keller; **14: Getty Images/**Catherine Ledner; **16: Mother & Baby Picture Library/**Ian Hooton; **18: Science Photo Library/**Lea Paterson; **20: Science Photo Library/**Manfred Kage; **28: Science Photo Library (tc), Science Photo Library/**John Walsh (tl); **29: Science Photo Library/**Zephyr; **31: The Wellcome Institute Library, London/**Yorgos Nikas; **34-35: Alamy Images/**David Young-Wolff; **37: Science Photo Library/**Edelmann (tr); **48: Alamy Images/**foodfolio; **51: Mother & Baby Picture Library/**Ian Hooton; **52: Mother & Baby Picture Library/**Ian Hooton; **56: Mother & Baby Picture Library/**Caroline Molloy; **57:** Laura Goetzl (tc, tr); **59: Science Photo Library/**CNRI (tr); **61: Science Photo Library/**Neil Bromhall; **67: Mother & Baby Picture Library; 69: Corbis/**RNT Productions; **71: Alamy Images/**David Young-Wolff; **73: Retna Pictures Ltd/**John Powell; **75: Getty Images/**gi Stock; **76: Mother & Baby Picture Library/**Ian Hooton; **79: Alamy Images/**Chad Ehlers; **81: Science Photo Library/**BSIP Laurent (bl); **82: Mother & Baby Picture Library/**Ian Hooton; **83: Science Photo Library/**GE Medical Systems; **86: Alamy Images/**eurekaimages.com; **89: Getty Images/**Ericka McConnell; **91: Zefa Visual Media/**J. Feingersh; **92-93: Mother & Baby Picture Library/**Ian Hooton; **94: Anthony Blake Photo Library/**Joy Skipper; **97: Science Photo Library/**Saturn Stills; **99: Mother & Baby Picture Library/**Ian Hooton; **101: Bubbles/**Chris Rout; **103: Alamy Images/**John Fortunato (br), **Science Photo Library/**Eye of Science (tl); **104: Alamy Images/**David Young-Wolff; **106: Corbis/**Anne W. Krause; **107: Alamy Images/**thislife pictures; **109: Science Photo Library; 112: Science Photo Library/**BSIP, Laurent; **113: Bubbles/**Frans Rombout; **115: Mother & Baby Picture Library/**Indira Flack; **117: Mother & Baby Picture Library/**Ruth Jenkinson; **122: Corbis/**Tom Stewart; **124: Mother & Baby Picture Library/**Ruth Jenkinson; **126: Mother & Baby Picture Library/**Paul Mitchell; **127: Mother & Baby Picture Library/**Eddie Lawrence; **128: Alamy Images/**Janine Wiedel (br); **130: Mother & Baby Picture Library/**Ruth Jenkinson; **132: Mother & Baby Picture Library/**Ruth Jenkinson; **133: Science Photo Library/**Ruth Jenkinson/ MIDIRS; **137: Mother & Baby Picture Library/**Frances Tout; **141: Photolibrary.com/**Mayer Eisenhut; **147: Corbis/**Larry Williams and Associates; **150: Mother & Baby Picture Library/**Ian Hooton.

All other images © Dorling Kindersley. For further information see **www.dkimages.com**

about the authors

Laura Goetzl MD MPH is a specialist in high-risk pregnancy who practises and teaches at the Medical University of South Carolina in Charleston, South Carolina. She is board certified in Obstetrics and Gynecology and Maternal–fetal Medicine, and is a member of the American College of Obstetrics and Gynecology, the Society for Maternal–fetal Medicine, and the American Institute of Ultrasound in Medicine. Dr. Goetzl balances her career with the demands of her husband's practice in surgical oncology. Together they care for their two small children, Gabriela and Lucas.

Regine Harford BS MS PhD is a medical writer with special interest in women's health. She is a member of the American Medical Writers Association and covers international medical conferences for the pharmaceutical industry, helps medical professionals with their publications and presentations, and brings up-to-date, relevant information to consumers. Giving birth to her youngest child at 39 provided her with first-hand experience of the joys and challenges of mature motherhood. Regine is based near Atlanta, Georgia.

authors' acknowledgments

Laura Goetzl:
I would like to thank my mentor, Joe Leigh Simpson MD, who first suggested this project to me. And most importantly my family, Nestor, Gabriela, and Lucas, who both supported and tolerated me during its completion.

Regine Harford:
Just as pregnancy and parenting challenges us as mothers, having a mom with a career can test the patience of our children. Therefore, I want to thank my sons, Markus, Christian, and Andrew, for supporting my work on this book, even during their summer break. You guys are the joy of my life!

From both authors:
A heartfelt thank you to the Pregnancy and Childcare team at Dorling Kindersley for helping us turn our initial efforts into the finished book you see today: to Jennifer Williams in the US; to Salima Hirani for conceiving and initiating this project; to Sara Kimmins and Alison Tumer for adding visual effect; and especially to Janet Mohun for accompanying us step-by-step through the writing process.

publisher's acknowledgments.

Dorling Kindersley would like to thank
Salima Hirani for her initial work in developing the concept for the book and for additional editorial assistance; Mrs Sarah Reynolds, consultant obstetrician and gynaecologist at the Bedford hospital, Bedford for reading the manuscript and ensuring the accuracy of UK specific information; Ruth Jenkinson for new photography; Sally Smallwood for organizing the photoshoots; Angela Baynham for editorial assistance; Mehmet Altun, Vijay Baldwin, Victoria Burns, Robin Brunson, Roshni Carter, Michelle Drew, Sarah Fairclough, Sarah Gardner, Dianna Harvey-Kummer, Rita Khosla-Wilson, and Joanna Stein for modelling; Hilary Bird for the index and Ann Baggaley for proofreading.